BREAST
CANCER

50

Essential Things You Can Do

BREAST CANCER

50

Essential Things You Can Do

GREG ANDERSON

Founder & CEO, Cancer Recovery Group

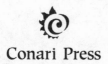

Conari Press

First published in 2011 by Conari Press, an imprint of
Red Wheel/Weiser, LLC
With offices at:
665 Third Street, Suite 400
San Francisco, CA 94107
www.redwheelweiser.com

Many of the characters in this book are composites of real people.
They are not intended to portray specific individuals unless named.

ISBN: 978-1-57324-536-4

Library of Congress Cataloging-in-Publication Data
is available on request.

Cover design by Nita Ybarra
Cover photograph © Austin Kulp/Cancer Recovery Group
Interior by Dutton & Sherman
Typeset in Goudy Old Style text and Palace Script, Requiem, and Serlio
Display

Printed in Canada
TCP
10 9 8 7 6 5 4 3 2 1

This book is dedicated to my wife, Linda.
Your unconditional loving sustains me.

Contents

Foreword

EVERY NOW AND THEN A BOOK comes along that truly resets the grid for how we think and how we behave. When it comes to breast cancer, this is one of those books. As I read through it, I kept thinking, *At LAST, a book that tells women with breast cancer—either newly diagnosed or with a recurrence—the whole truth. On every level—body, mind, and spirit. And then gives them a concrete way to access their own healing power. Eureka!*

So many things are right about this book. First and foremost, Greg Anderson knows exactly what he's talking about. He has personally helped over 19,000 individuals design their best integrative treatment plans that incorporate social supports, nutrition, massage, meditation, and other approaches to their care that involve their whole being, their person, and not just their disease. He has been there himself. Diagnosed with terminal lung cancer many years ago, Greg accessed his inner ability to heal, has been cancer free for decades, and now teaches others what he has learned.

Interestingly enough, lung cancer—like breast cancer—occurs in the area of the fourth chakra, commonly known as the heart chakra, the part of the body most closely associated with giving and receiving whole-heartedly, releasing grief and resentment, and allowing in full partnership and joy. This similarity tells us that Greg knows very intimately the kind of emotional healing that is required for those who have breast cancer.

There's another important point I want to stress about this book. It could not have been written by a doctor who treats breast cancer. Why? Because the practice of medicine is overly focused on drugs and surgery, and the belief system that runs conventional medicine is that the tumor (or the germ) is the enemy, and the enemy must be eliminated by any means possible, however toxic. This belief is so engrained in current medical practice that to step outside and suggest other treatments is to risk professional censure or even the loss of one's license or hospital privileges.

In conventional medicine, the body's innate ability to heal itself is virtually ignored. And the role of nutrition in general and vitamin D in particular are misunderstood or simply not addressed. I recall very vividly that back in the early 1980's, when I'd counsel a breast cancer patient about her diet, I'd have to close my door so that my colleagues wouldn't hear me engaging in what was, at that time, medical heresy. Yes, just diet! That might surprise you, given that nutrition is more widely accepted as a legitimate science now. (Which is not to say that an institutional medical bias against it doesn't remain.)

Yet it is still entirely too perilous for a doctor to talk to a patient about the role of her emotions and her relationships in her state of health. It is still taboo to stand at the bedside of a breast cancer patient and suggest that her cancer may, in part, be associated with an unmet need for nurturance or for expressing a loss that has not been acknowledged. This is considered "blaming the victim," because doctors are simply not taught how to deal with their own emotions, let alone those of their patients.

This fear of victim blaming keeps doctors from even mentioning the role of the human spirit and emotions in diseases like cancer. I'm not suggesting that anyone should be *blamed* for becoming ill. But that doesn't mean we should deny that disease has emotional links and that working through difficult emotional material is a critical component of healing. This "keep emotion out of it" mindset that pervades the teaching and practice of medicine robs us of our true power to heal—by pointing us in the opposite direction of where true healing lies.

Clearly there is nothing to be gained by a stance that includes blame in any way. And one must have a relationship with her healthcare practitioner that is based on empathy and compassion before it feels safe to uncover emotions as uncomfortable as guilt, shame, resentment, or anger. But the first step in the healing process is validation of the role of emotions in the first place! As Marshall Rosenberg so brilliantly points out in his work on nonviolent communication (*www.cnvc.org*), our emotions are designed to help us get our needs met. Unfortunately, many of us have been shamed or blamed for having legitimate needs from early childhood. This includes the need for enough sleep, recognition, love, touch, and so on. Unmet and invalidated childhood needs can stay locked in our bodies for years, with each producing an overabundance of stress hormones. These stress hormones, in turn, set the stage for later disease.

The famous ACE (Adverse Childhood Experiences) study from Kaiser Permanente provides very powerful documentation of how unmet childhood needs set the stage for illness. This study found that adverse childhood experiences are vastly more common than is recognized or acknowledged—and they often map directly to disease. Slightly more than half of the 17,000 middle-class, middle-aged study participants in the ACE study had grown up in dysfunctional alcoholic homes, homes with a depressed or mentally ill person, or homes in which they had experienced sexual, physical, or emotional abuse. These individuals, with unmet needs for things as basic as physical safety, were far more likely to incur greater pharmacy costs, doctor visits, emergency room visits, hospitalization, and premature death.

The ACE study certainly validated my own clinical experience. Back in the early 1980's I found that nearly every woman who came to see me with severe PMS, for example, had come from a home in which alcohol, mental illness, or other dysfunction was present. Severe PMS—as well as most other illness to some degree—results from the biochemical effect of chronic stress and subsequent poor lifestyle choices. I've often been reminded of the observation of Lewis Thomas, the former director of the Memorial Sloan Kettering Cancer Center in New York, who wrote, "I have come to believe that cancer is the physical metaphor for the extreme need to grow."

Not surprisingly, those doctors who are brave enough to mention the role of emotions in healing and also tell the whole truth about overtreatment often face the censure and criticism of their colleagues. Because Greg is not a medical insider, he is free to tell the whole truth about things that most doctors are reluctant to admit. One of those truths is that breast cancer is often drastically overtreated in ways that can adversely affect a woman for the rest of her life. Lymphedema of the arm and radiation damage to the heart and lungs instantly come to mind. Anderson fearlessly—and compassionately—takes the time to explain why and how this sort of overtreatment is allowed to happen. For example, he explains how the bone marrow transplant—a brutal treatment—came to be accepted as the standard of care for certain kinds of breast cancer back in the 1990's despite inadequate data on its efficacy. (I had a number of patients barely survive the treatment itself.) He also tells the truth about the political maneuverings that got the insurance companies to cover it and other undertested and often health-threatening treatments.

In short, the information in this book is not only groundbreaking and eye-opening, it is also galvanizing and life-saving. Hear this: *Breast Cancer: 50 Essential Things You Can Do* needs to be in the hands of every woman who has been diagnosed with breast cancer— or who is afraid that she will be. Bravo, Greg Anderson.

Christiane Northrup, MD

Getting the Most from This Book

THIS IS MORE THAN A BOOK. It is a life-saving guide, a roadmap for women on the journey through breast cancer. The message will enable you to discover the answer to the two most important questions: How can I get well? How can I stay well?

By the end of this journey, you will know and understand the big picture—how all these pathways converge, coming together to synergistically contribute to fighting illness and creating new levels of health and well-being.

Through our work at Breast Cancer Charities of America, we have come to observe and understand that the majority of women who not only survive but also thrive following a breast cancer diagnosis exhibit many or all of the following characteristics:

First and foremost, they come to the deep belief in their body's ability to heal. Note the emphasis; the belief is about the body healing, not about the cancer being treated. This is a crucial point of understanding. This theme is revisited again and again in this book.

These same women regain a sense of control over their lives—a sense that leads to assuming personal accountability for creating a breast cancer recovery program that is uniquely right for them. These heroines do not passively hand over responsibility to their doctors and expect a miracle. They proactively fight.

Many survivors also undergo what we have come to describe as a spiritual awakening, becoming vividly aware of and then honoring the long-dormant values and aspirations they have long suppressed. This reawakening—being truly mindful, perhaps for the first time—

brings a new authenticity to their lives. Many look back on breast cancer as a gift that helped them in this transformation.

These same women fully reassess their lives, often becoming relationship sensitive, distancing themselves especially from people to whom they formerly felt beholden. Work and career changes are common as these women release their passion and energy toward what matters most.

Healthy lifestyle choices take center stage with an emphasis on wise nutrition. These women shift away from refined and processed foods. They move toward plant-based diets, consuming more vegetables and fruit and fewer unhealthy fats. And they take vitamin and mineral supplements to help support immune health.

Daily exercise is simply part of this new lifestyle. Survivors move. They consider the exercise discipline a fundamental component of staying well. Importantly, they find a physical activity that generates joy. Exercise becomes a "get to," not a "have to."

These disciplines are balanced with a greater awareness of taking time—making time—to relax and enjoy life. The need for play is honored. And for many, meditation and prayer become important parts of daily life.

Survivors release guilt. They forgive—themselves and others. They find the ability to love without condition, and this factor alone creates a life experience that optimally supports health.

And finally, breast cancer survivors tend to become more aware of community, connecting with and reclaiming the sense of a life filled with meaning and purpose that comes from being of service to others, often other breast cancer patients.

This is what I wish for you. Come alive. Using the guidance in this book, I encourage you to become fully engaged in your own health and healing. The aim here is to present you and those you love with a better, more natural, and ultimately holistic way of traveling the breast cancer journey.

Treat the illness? Yes. Appropriate, minimally invasive, least toxic medical treatment has its place.

But even more, create health—physically, emotionally, and even spiritually. When you do, you will not only improve your physical well-being, you will also improve your life.

Erica A. Harvey
Founder and Executive Director
Breast Cancer Charities of America and the iGoPink Campaign

Preface

THE BREAST CANCER JOURNEY is a long and winding road, the ultimate uncertain pathway of vulnerability. Challenges lie at every twist and turn. There seems to be a shortage of unbiased maps.

Although few would choose this journey, the experience is inevitably profound. At its worst, breast cancer may seem like it can destroy body, mind, and spirit. At its best, breast cancer is a journey of discovery that yields new levels of personal wisdom, strength, and dignity.

When traveled with grace, with an open mind and spirit, the breast cancer journey can lead to a deeper understanding of what it means to be a woman, and it can even reveal one's unique role in the world.

You are now on this incredible journey. I know in my heart that you can travel this winding path successfully. I am here to help you do so.

I will assume you are reading this book because you are in one of two positions. You are either:

- A breast cancer patient
- Supporting a friend or loved one who is dealing with breast cancer

If this describes you, I ask you to read the next sentence very carefully:

Your goal is to create health and well-being—physically, emotionally, and spiritually—not simply to treat the tumor.

For more than a quarter century after I received a terminal lung cancer diagnosis, my life's mission has been to offer help, hope, and healing to people experiencing cancer. With my wife, Linda, and the Cancer Recovery Group, we extend that same offer to the loved ones who support cancer patients. The most frequent type of diagnosis we deal with is breast cancer.

The essential focus of the work is to offer patients a program that unlocks their inherent ability to heal, to create health. We help patients learn about and use their body's significant self-healing resources to live healthier, richer, and longer lives. While there is no natural approach that can guarantee the curing of breast cancer by itself, there is extensive evidence to show that the many things you can do to support your own healing are at least as important as the conventional medical treatments offered by orthodox oncology.

You have an astonishing ability. You possess the ability to heal. You carry within you a healing intelligence that transcends mere medicine. For example, perhaps you accidentally cut yourself. The wound is deep and long. Within moments you find yourself on the way to the emergency room. The wound is cleaned and sutured. You are told to check with your family practitioner.

Provided the bandages are periodically changed and the wound is kept clean, healing proceeds. You do not have to do a thing. Six weeks later, your doctor says all is well.

Did the emergency room physician who sutured your wound accomplish your healing? No. She simply secured the severed tissue. Is your family doctor to be credited with your healing? No, he simply helped you keep the wound clean. Your medical team may have treated you, but something on a higher level accomplished the healing.

You healed. The astonishing inner healing intelligence you possess is to be credited. The good news is that this intelligence awaits your discovery in your journey through breast cancer.

In this book, I am going to do everything possible to encourage you to consciously embrace what I have come to call your Inner Healer. Your active participation with this power is some of the most important work in which you have ever engaged.

Breast Cancer: 50 Essential Things You Can Do is written for those people who want to survive the experience of cancer and who are willing to participate actively in the recovery process. This book's goal is twofold: to inform you on the major issues following a breast cancer diagnosis and to encourage you to implement a comprehensive recovery plan of your design that has your highest confidence level.

This program is designed to help you maximize your opportunity for a complete recovery while maintaining a high quality of life. This is not a book to be read and then put away, never to be referred to again. Instead, think of using this as your health and healing resource guide for the next two years—a reasonable time for recovery. Return to it again and again for periodic checkups or to get "unstuck" in your breast cancer journey.

I believe this book has a meaningful message for every person affected by breast cancer. The strategies are tailor-made for the person with a new diagnosis. If you have recently been told, "You have breast cancer," you'll find here the information you need to gain control over your fears, analyze your diagnosis, and put in place the most effective integrated cancer care program possible. For the newly diagnosed, I recommend following the 50 Essential Things You Can Do (see chapter 7) in order. There is a certain logical progression in their sequence. You need a plan. Here it is. Following this pattern will prove invaluable and will ensure that you are making the wisest decisions possible.

This book is also written for the person who has been diagnosed with a recurrence of breast cancer. Recurrence is often a frightening event, a time of medical reevaluation as well as a physical, emotional, and spiritual turning point. I encourage you to make the 50 Essential Things the very heart of your entire analysis. Thoughtfully follow the steps. Use this book as your primary guide. A recurrence does not equate with death. What you do does make a difference. See the 50 Essential Things You Can Do as mandatory points of action. Then you'll know you're doing everything possible to regain your good health.

Before you begin reading, secure a notebook and a pen, or create a new folder on your laptop. I want you to create a Wellness and Recovery Journal. I started mine with a single sheet of my daughter's notebook paper and an old three-ring binder. Nothing elaborate is required. As you read, questions and insights will come to mind. Record them. You'll find yourself clipping newspaper and magazine articles about cancer. Tape them into your notebook. This is going to become your primary source book, a reference manual for your personal referral. Now, twenty-seven years after I was told I would die, I have many binders harboring a wealth of insights that are important to me. I still add information. My journal also serves as an excellent log recording my cancer recovery journey.

Please do the same. You need the clarity the Wellness and Recovery Journal delivers. Even though a road map to recovery is contained in this book, each person must ultimately chart his or her own course.

Use your Wellness and Recovery Journal to record your unique personal insights. Especially record your questions. Then ask. Ask your doctor, your medical technicians, and other survivors. Nothing is to be assumed. Ask about medical terms that you don't understand. Ask about reasons for tests. Ask about the results of those tests. Ask for success stories. Ask. Ask. Ask.

Asking questions gives you significant power. Do not be intimidated by medical jargon, healthcare providers, or the diagnostic and treatment process. You are the one in charge. Ask! Then record the responses. Come back to them again and again.

Through this entire journey, there is good reason to be filled with hope, provided you take an active part in the recovery process. Understand this recurring theme: you must not passively treat illness; you must actively create health. Join me. Let's get started.

The Woodlands, Texas
Spring 2011

Acknowledgments

A HEARTFELT THANK-YOU TO ALL my friends and colleagues at Cancer Recovery Group. I treasure you.

A sincere thank you to my editor, Caroline Pincus. You repeatedly encouraged me to address the issue of breast cancer. Your skill in bringing this message to fruition is unparalleled. Thank you, my friend and colleague.

Several pioneers in integrated cancer care need to be recognized. The late O. Carl Simonton, MD, is the father of modern psychosocial oncology. His work yielded consistent evidence that mind-body techniques such as relaxation, self-hypnosis, and guided imagery significantly reduce stress and anxiety in cancer patients and contribute to recovery.

In Canada, Alastair Cunningham, PhD, traced substantial improvements in quality of life for those cancer patients who adopted the holistic strategy. His work also confirms the validity of the growing body of evidence that psychospiritual self-help not only prolongs life but is also correlated with unexpected remissions of cancer.

I wish to recognize the work of Cedric Garland and the late Frank Garland, both epidemiologists associated with the University of California at San Diego. They established the link between vitamin D deficiency and breast cancer. They were the first to note higher breast cancer incidence in the northern latitudes, where sunlight is noticeably lower than, for instance, in the Southwestern United States. It is their work that led Cancer Recovery Group to be the first public health agency to issue recommendations for vitamin D supplementation for cancer prevention.

My highest respect to Sad Dharam Kaur, ND, for the meticulous work in researching and documenting the wealth of science that validates the power of the natural healing methods referenced throughout this book.

I wish to recognize Dr. Hal Gunn and his entire team at Inspire-Health in Vancouver, British Columbia. You have implemented the world's preeminent model of integrated cancer care. Thank you for your kindness in allowing me to share your work with a broader audience.

To all who so generously gave their time, talents, and creativity to this project, please accept my sincere appreciation.

And to all who search these pages for the answers to wellness, my encouragement and my love.

Author's Note

THE IDEAS IN THIS BOOK are meant to supplement the care and guidance of competent medical professionals. At no time does the author suggest that these steps take the place of conventional medical treatment. Do not attempt a self-diagnosis. Do not embark upon self-treatment of a serious illness without professional help. There are a growing number of informed doctors who will work with their clients to integrate body, mind, and spirit. Find one. Form a healing partnership.

Part One

Understanding the Incredible Journey

The Emerging Model of Breast Cancer Care

I T'S NOT ALL ABOUT THE TREATMENT.
    Several years ago, I received a call from Ruth, a medical doctor who was part of a family practice based near Chicago, Illinois. About two years earlier, she was diagnosed with breast cancer. Things were not going well. "I need other options," she said.

As we talked, Ruth first shared how she'd recently become exceedingly depressed and quit her work to have time to heal. However, she was now stuck, overwhelmed by the thought that she may not live to see her two children become adults. She hoped I might share with her more details of the recent findings I'd reported at a conference she'd attended.

From the perspective of orthodox medicine, Ruth was strictly following protocol, doing everything perfectly. This included a mastectomy followed by both chemotherapy and radiation. She'd recently switched from tamoxifen to raloxifene because the reduced risks of adverse effects, especially blood clots, seemed to dictate that change to her. After talking for about twenty minutes, Ruth agreed to complete the Cancer Recovery Group's standard intake form and email it back to me. A follow-up appointment was set for two weeks.

Except for too much refined sugar in her diet, Ruth's responses to our questionnaire were standard. Our second phone call was anything but.

She first needed to talk about her surgeon, a man to whom she had often referred her own patients. They were professional colleagues, and their spouses even knew one another, she told me. Then Ruth angrily and tearfully unloaded.

"After my diagnosis was confirmed," said Ruth, "our entire relationship changed. Now I was told exactly what to do, to share the intimate details of my life, to describe my symptoms and even my monthly menstrual cycles and private sexual behavior. I was stripped naked, both physically and emotionally. I was just another patient. I saw the privileged status of doctor ripped away from me. To the medical system, I was now reduced to just another Stage II infiltrating ductal carcinoma. I was expected to do as I was told. And beyond genetic mutations, my doctors could provide no insights into why I contracted this god-awful disease."

The Question of Cause

There is no one cause for all breast cancers. Nor is there just one treatment for all breast cancers. Many factors contribute to cancer development, and many factors help prevent its development. This includes diet, exercise, toxin exposure, vitamin D levels, hormones, certain medical tests and treatments, as well as gender, age, genetics, race, and more. These factors, interacting together, impact breast cancer development and prevention. For each woman, the combination will be different. The emerging model of breast care recognizes this complexity.

In a sense, Ruth's doctors were correct. On the cellular level, breast cancer is an expression of genes that have mutated, resulting in cells that have gone awry. But bad genetics are not the cause of 90 to 95 percent of breast cancers. An unlucky draw from the genetic pool explains just 5 to 10 percent of the factors involved in the development of breast cancer.

Genes gone bad are actually the result, the outcome, of many other factors. Your genes turn off and on in relation to the environment in which those genes live. The good news is that even if we do have a gene that potentially predisposes us to cancer development, lifestyle factors can and will impact the degree to which that gene is expressed.

Dr. Dean Ornish, one of the world's most esteemed pioneers and integrated healthcare revolutionaries, stated, "People should realize that genes may be our predisposition, but they are not our fate. The fact is, massive positive changes in genetic activity are generated through lifestyle choices. Our choices are as powerful as our strongest drugs and occur rapidly in most individuals."

How powerful? Among the researchers who study lifestyle's impact on health, there is a consensus that 50 to 75 percent of cancers are totally and completely preventable. Excellent and compelling scientific evidence shows that eight of ten breast cancers could be prevented, actually stopped before diagnosis. I ask you to pause to consider these points for just a moment. Isn't that a startling revelation?

There's more. Prevention can be accomplished by minimizing or eliminating factors that predispose one to cancer development. These include reducing the consumption of animal fats, avoiding inactivity, eliminating the use of tobacco, and moderating the consumption of alcohol. Prevention of breast cancer is also accomplished by adding nutritional supplements that reduce genetic expression. We will have much more to say about this later in the book.

There's even more good news. If breast cancer can be prevented through these measures, common sense tells us that these same healthful self-care measures will also be of value in both the recovery process and in reducing the risk of recurrence. Happily, there is excellent emerging science to support the huge role that self-care plays in recovery.

There is significant resistance to these natural-healing ideas in much of the orthodox oncology community. Even though Hippocrates, the father of modern medicine, said, more than 2,500 years ago, "Let food be thy medicine and thy medicine thy food," many Western-trained doctors have little tolerance for such ideas. "Eat whatever you want" is what both my surgeon and my radiation oncologist told me. They were more concerned that I ate any-thing and everything, sugars and fats included, in order to keep my weight up.

Like most of us, doctors are busy people. Most do their very best to keep apprised of everything that is going on in their field. The good ones constantly read new scientific studies published in professional journals, attend conferences, and see pharmaceutical representatives several times a year. But as a result, there is a perva-sive attitude that says, "If it were true, I would know about it." But clearly, this is an incorrect assumption, especially when it comes to more natural approaches to breast cancer.

Nutrition, exercise, social support, and mind/body/spirit matters are barely, if ever, on the curriculum in medical school. Following a talk I gave at the world-famous MD Anderson Cancer Center in Houston, Texas, a medical oncologist pulled me aside and said, "You must stop spreading these unfounded statements about diet." She went on to insist that double-blind studies were the gold standard by which to measure all cancer interventions. This is an accurate illustration of the state of mind in which most doctors live and work. There is a profound medical culture bias that dismisses natural approaches in favor of pharmaceutical solutions. She concluded by saying, "Patients don't want to change what they eat. And they sure don't want to exercise. They want to receive their treatment and then forget about it."

Some oncologists have also said to me, "Even if we lower the [research] standards, you experts can't even agree among yourselves. There's just no consensus in the natural health field." My response was that patients should do everything possible to help prevent and control cancer in ways that do not harm the body. Predictably, I was asked to provide proof there would be no harm. The demand for hard science stands in the way of common sense—it's the state of oncology in America and much of the world today.

That said, it is important to note that people who exercise regu-larly and eat healthfully can still develop breast cancer. Remember, breast cancer is not a single-cause disease. And for each person, the combination of causative factors is different. However, we can all learn to take better care of ourselves physically, emotionally, and spiritually. A diagnosis of breast cancer is the signal to do so, providing an opportunity to fully love and care for oneself. That truth stands as the premier attribute of the emerging model of breast care.

The History

Conventional Western breast cancer treatment is exclusively focused on the disease. It's the tumor model. Following a myriad of tests, a diagnosis is made. Once diagnosed, the tumor or the blood-based cancer is attacked with surgery, chemotherapy, and/or radiation. Medical expertise is required to prescribe and administer these treatments, and thus a different specialist is necessary to implement each treatment type. The entire process is all about the tumor and precious little about the person.

For Ruth, walking through the gates and into the cancer treatment terrain started poorly. Prior to her initial surgery, she was told she needed a CT scan to determine if the tumor had attached to the chest wall. Ruth knew CT scans were not routinely used in a Stage II breast cancer diagnosis. But the surgeon was insistent. He said, "I need to know whether or not the tumor can be removed with mastectomy." Reluctantly, Ruth agreed.

The test did not go well. CT scans, also called CAT scans or computed tomography scans, require a dye, which acts as a contrast solution, be injected into your arm through an intravenous line prior to the test. "The technician who tried to insert the IV," said Ruth, "knew not what the hell he was doing. First, he couldn't find a vein. Then he dropped the entire IV kit on the floor. Instead of throwing it away and securing a new one, he picked it up and was about to use this now unsterile apparatus on me. I yelled at him, 'Stop it!' And I walked out the door.

"He didn't know who I was," continued Ruth. "He cared only about the procedure and nothing about me, his patient. There I sat in that god-awful gown in that cold exam room, afforded no human comfort, no respect, and no acknowledgment that I was a living and breathing human being let alone a medical professional. At that moment, I had this sinking feeling. I realized the system in which I was trained, and in which I practiced, would eventually fail me."

Breast cancer patients most often turn to the Cancer Recovery Group after the system has in some way failed them. Perhaps these women are concerned about the tests used to arrive at their diagnosis. Or they feel as if they are being rushed, even forced, into treatments without understanding their options. Many breast cancer patients reach out to us only after traditional medical treatments have failed and they've heard the frightening words "Your cancer is back."

Overtreatment

Much too often, these brave women turn to us when they are physically so weak and fragile that they fear they can withstand no more treatment. "Radiation has me so fatigued I can't function," they say. Or "I cannot go through another round of chemotherapy." The sad fact is we spend a great deal of time and effort helping cancer patients deal with overtreatment.

I first became vividly aware of the problem of overtreatment in the early 1990s. A young California mother by the name of Nelene Fox turned to us for guidance. She had an advanced invasive ductal carcinoma. Her first words were surprising: "Can you help me raise the $250,000 I need for a bone marrow transplant?" Her insurance provider, Health Net, refused to cover the procedure because they considered it unproven and experimental.

Those were brutal days in breast cancer treatment. Oncologists boldly proclaimed that high-dose chemotherapy followed by bone marrow transplant offered the cure for advanced breast cancer. And medical journalists, especially in the major weekly news magazines, blindly fanned the flames of this optimism. Many in the breast cancer community proclaimed high-dose chemo and bone marrow transplant to be the Holy Grail.

The procedure was exceedingly dangerous. I retain a newspaper clipping in which one doctor describes the process. "We bring the patient to death's door through an intensive pretransplant regimen of chemotherapy and radiation. Our treatment involves a four-drug regimen and is 35 to 40 percent more intensive than the regimens used in the recently reported studies. We administer our regimen in a highly specialized transplant unit, not in the outpatient setting. Although the treatment itself is associated with a 21 percent mortality rate, the payoff may be a higher proportion of women surviving and being cancer free." Brutal by any standards.

While trying to persuade Health Net to pay for the bone marrow transplant, Nelene Fox did raise the funds to have the procedure. But eight months later, she died. Her brother, Mark Hiepler, is an attorney, and he brought a lawsuit against his sister's insurance company. He won, and the jury awarded the Fox family $89 million. Although the settlement was subsequently negotiated down to smaller sum, the case is considered a watershed moment in that thereafter most health insurance companies began approving high-dose chemotherapy with bone marrow transplant for advanced breast cancer.

This era spawned a desperate flurry of activities attempting to position this procedure as the quintessential answer to breast cancer. With the financial help of the biggest international pharmaceutical companies including Amgen, Aventis, Pharmacia, and Wyeth, the procedure was researched and promoted. Transplant doctors testified before Congress and appeared in the media. Breast cancer advocacy groups like the Susan G. Komen Breast Cancer Foundation, now called Susan G. Komen for the Cure, lobbied both federal authorities and state legislatures to mandate insurance coverage for the procedure. Hospitals from coast to coast proudly rushed to equip their facilities with bone marrow transplant units, encouraging their physicians to learn the procedure. Providing transplants for breast cancer patients was good business.

At that time, the Cancer Recovery Group was based in Southern California, where we ran the largest cancer support group in the nation. We always built our message around less toxic and least invasive prevention and treatment options. But in the early 1990s, our message was drowned out. For nearly five years, the number one request from patients and their family members was information on high-dose chemo and bone marrow transplant.

New drugs were introduced that made it possible to harvest marrow cells from blood rather than having to extract it from a woman's hip. And soon it was possible to administer high-dose chemo and transplant on an outpatient basis. It was all systems go to make high-dose chemotherapy and bone marrow transplant the new standard of care. Its efficacy was accepted as an article of faith.

It wasn't until 1999 at an American Society of Clinical Oncology (ASCO) meeting that researchers presented four studies that showed women did no better with the high-dose chemotherapy and bone marrow transplant treatment than those who received only low-dose chemotherapy. From that point forward, the procedure was discredited and today is largely abandoned.

More Is Not Better

The beliefs behind the more-treatment mindset die hard and are the reason so much unnecessary care is still delivered by doctors and hospitals. In the world of breast cancer care, it is widely agreed that surgery is the most effective treatment, contributing more to halting the progression of the disease than the other treatment modalities combined. Yet beyond surgery, there is little certainty about which drugs or which procedures actually work best.

Our culture seeks cures. Most people in developed societies believe fervently in the doctrine that modern medicine cures. Cure—it's almost a statement of faith, pervasive on every continent. And most breast cancer patients look to its high priests, the oncologists, as their saviors. We seldom question the ongoing march of science. In fact, we expect it, taking scientific progress as a given. Both patients and healthcare professionals are deeply in need of believing that medicine cures.

That belief fosters a more-treatment-is-better-treatment senti-ment that is deeply imbedded in conventional Western oncology. It is driven by physician-specialists who don't really know which of the major treatment modalities are truly the most effective. It leads to massive overtreatment.

This is exacerbated by the hammer syndrome, something I first explored more than twenty years ago. The syndrome looks like this: If you are a surgeon, every answer looks like surgery. If you are a radi-ation oncologist, all your answers point toward radiation. And if you are a medical oncologist, every answer involves drugs. I'll have more to say about chemotherapy later. The point is, if you are trained in a narrow subspecialty, that's what you see as the answer. If you're a hammer, the whole world looks like a nail.

But there is much more to this overtreatment warning. Most oncologists lack the specialized training needed to independently interpret the evidence that is available to them. This leads even well-intentioned physicians to treat patients out of an understand-able altruistic and humanitarian motive to help, even when they may not know what is the best thing to do.

Medical oncologists are famous for statements like "We will never know if this drug can help you unless we do just one more round." There is a vast array of evidence that suggests the last round is often the fatal round. The Cancer Recovery Group's work has led me to believe that thousands of patients die each year not from cancer but from cancer treatment.

In the mid-1990s, my wife and I personally walked through a breast cancer experience with Denise, a close family friend. I knew virtually all the members of the medical team, including the medical oncologist. After he delivered Denise's diagnosis and reviewed the recommended treatment protocol, the kindly, soft-spoken, and well-meaning oncologist pulled me aside and said, "Your friend is in for a rough time. We can give her a year, maybe a little more."

Denise and her family had blind faith in medicine. We asked, "What are the other treatment options?" The answer was some early-stage clinical trials. I tried to explain the dangers of early-stage clinical trials. But Denise's answer was always "Let's try." At the end of her battle, the kindly doctor called me to say, "We tried this new drug. It's a shot in the dark. But we'll never know unless we try." Denise never made it out of the hospital alive, another victim of overtreatment.

In America, the fear of malpractice drives what is euphemistically called defensive medicine. This is the practice of diagnostic and therapeutic procedures conducted primarily as a safeguard against possible malpractice liability, not as a means to improve a patient's health. In breast cancer, fear of litigation is often behind a long list of diagnostic scans, genetic tests, specialty surgeries, and treatment recommendations involving radiation and chemotherapy even when the cancer has been diagnosed at the very earliest stages.

Overtreatment may also be due to prevailing local medical practices. Even when excellent outcome-based evidence exists, treatment choices can and do vary dramatically from place to place.

This is clearly the case in early-stage breast cancer. Studies show that mastectomy and lumpectomy achieve similar long-term survival. But doctors differ sharply in their attitudes toward these treatments. John E. Wennberg, MD, MPH, pointed out in his Dartmouth Atlas studies that there are regions in the United States in which virtually no Medicare women underwent lumpectomy, while in another, nearly half did.

Why such massive disparity? Clearly, it was not based on science, as the studies show similar outcomes. Based on science, you could expect something closer to 50 percent mastectomies and 50 percent lumpectomies. But many treatment decisions are based on the notion of "That's the way we do it here." As a breast cancer patient, it is critical that you understand if local customs, rather than the best medicine, are driving your treatment recommendations. We'll cover the outcome-based treatment guidelines later in this book for your comparison and analysis.

Such extreme variations arise because patients commonly and willingly delegate decision making to their physicians. Decision delegation is most often given under the assumption that the doctor knows best. Behind it is a belief that physicians can always understand a patient's values and thus recommend the most appropriate treatment for each person. But often, very often, local custom rather than outcomes-based evidence drives these treatment recommendations. Studies show that when patients are fully informed about their options, they often choose very differently from their physicians.

Beyond all these very understandable reasons, I have come to believe that the most powerful reason American doctors and hospitals overtest and overtreat is that most of them are paid for how much care they deliver rather than how well they take care of their patients. Western medicine, especially as practiced in the United States, is reimbursed on a piece-rate basis. It's like the man on the old-fashioned assembly line: the more widgets he made, the more he was paid. This one factor alone has led to a massive overtreatment of many illnesses, including cancer, and especially breast and prostate cancers.

As is so often the case, it all comes down to the money. Harsh, I know, but true.

Hospitals, doctors, medical equipment manufacturers, pharmaceutical companies, and all the organizations that support breast cancer diagnosis and treatment have a bias. They have a deeply vested interest in the more-treatment-is-better-treatment paradigm. Pharmaceutical companies do not want medical oncologists to prescribe less chemotherapy. Manufacturers of radiology equipment do not promote the use of less radiation. And the companies that manufacture surgical gloves do not want fewer surgeries. It goes on and on and on.

Therefore, as you set foot on the breast cancer journey, be very aware. You are not looking for more medicine. You are seeking the best medicine. The two are not the same. This book will guide you in that quest.

The Shift

Because the focus of the tumor-based cancer care model is simply on the tumor, little if any effort is expended in exploring the benefits of healthful diet, regular exercise, immune-enhancing treatments, social and emotional support, spirituality, or other methods to enhance a patient's well-being. And as so often happens, a focus solely on the tumor leaves the thinking patient disempowered and unable to contribute to her own healing.

Let's be clear: surgery, chemotherapy, and radiation can play an important role in cancer treatment. But with breast cancer, especially early-stage breast cancer, the benefits that conventional treatment may provide must be carefully weighed against the risks. Those risks are great, including the potential for premature death and greatly reduced quality of life.

Conventional treatments do not address the underlying factors that prevent or predispose one to cancer development. Conventional breast cancer treatments treat symptoms. This includes the tumor. The tumor model of breast cancer care considers the tumor the entire problem. The emerging model of breast cancer treatment recognizes the tumor as a physical indication of a greater underlying imbalance.

Let's repeat: the new model of breast care recognizes the growing evidence that supporting and creating high levels of well-being with healthful nutrition and exercise are at least as important as any conventional cancer treatment. Plus, the broader aspects of emotional, social, and spiritual support can be critically important to creating optimal health and a level of well-being that transcends disease.

Science is beginning to discover what healers have known for centuries—that our mind and body and spirit are inseparable. Together they create a life force that nurtures health, healing, and the optimal functioning of our immune system. This means that health is much more than healthcare, that breast cancer is much more than breast cancer treatments.

Understanding and acknowledging that our body and mind and spirit are inseparable, the emerging paradigm of breast care provides optimal support for one's whole person. These disciplines can be naturally and safely integrated with conventional breast cancer treatments. Supporting overall health supports immune function, which in turn facilitates the healing process, improves our quality of life, and enhances recovery. In short, the wise integration of body, mind, and spirit creates health.

With the growing scientific evidence supporting this philosophy and these practices, the integrated approach is now embraced by an ever-increasing number of women diagnosed with breast cancer. Even a growing cadre of physicians, practitioners, and allied health-care professionals are coming forward to serve breast cancer patients in optimally engaging in their own health and healing. Unlike the early 1990s, today there is room for optimism.

The study of the relationship between the mind, body, and immune system is called psychoneuroimmunology. Scientists are discovering that when we feel empowered, our immune system is empowered. Fear can have a substantial negative impact on immune function, whereas regaining a sense of control and positive engagement in our own health and healing helps support immune function. The important principles of empowerment, self-engagement, and personal choice are at the heart of the emerging model of breast care.

More than any other dynamic, the emerging model understands that mind, body, spirit, and immune system are one. We are moving away from the single-dimension tumor model of breast cancer care toward multiple ways of supporting mind, body, spirit, and immune function, such as exercise, nutrition, and stress reduction. They are all interrelated, each contributing to the benefit provided by the others in a synergistic way. By engaging in the many ways we can support mind, body, and spirit, we clearly optimize our body's healing potential. And today we can say with certainty that a breast cancer recovery program without integration of body, mind, and spirit is incomplete.

Thousands of cases of recovery from so-called incurable, life-threatening diseases, including advanced cancers, have been scientifically documented. I am one of those documented cases. You also have that potential.

While research of this remarkable phenomenon is still in its infancy, we are now beginning to understand how we can more optimally support our body's amazing ability to heal. With growing scientific interest in this field, researchers have begun to study patients who have recovered in hopes of understanding how we all can better facilitate our body's remarkable healing abilities. And while that research is good and even necessary, I am asking you to act now to design and implement your own integrated breast cancer recovery program. There's simply no good reason to wait.

Beyond the Cause: Your Response

The new model of breast health means there is limited room for patient passivity. The patients who do well actively participate in creating health and well-being. The good news is that when we do engage in our own process of recovery, we regain a sense of autonomy, a feeling that we can impact our own health and life, a sense of being in charge. Numerous studies have shown that patients who become actively involved in designing their recovery plan are more likely to follow through with their treatments, less likely to have complications, and more likely to have favorable outcomes than those who simply take a passive role.

I do realize that becoming an active patient has its own challenges. Being told that you have breast cancer is usually a very frightening experience. Due to the technical nature of conventional cancer treatment regimens, those decisions tend to be driven by specialists. At this point, patients often become passive bystanders in their own care. Overwhelmed by procedures, treatments, and side effects that they may not understand, they acquiesce.

Most breast cancer patients are also haunted by questions about their prediagnosis role. I often hear statements like "Why me? What did I do wrong? What could I have done differently? Am I to blame for my breast cancer?" These questions are a natural response to a significant diagnosis. While natural, they can generate thoughts and feelings of worry, despair, self-blame, and even resentment toward others. Misunderstanding one's role very often adds further stress to an already challenging situation.

As a consequence, women with breast cancer are often left feeling isolated, frightened, and depressed, a state that inhibits both immune function and healing. In this context, patients may believe they are unable to contribute in a meaningful way to their recovery and, as a result, experience a sense of loss of control over their own health. At the very time an active response is called for, a passive reaction may be all that is forthcoming.

In our work, we help cancer patients reframe their experience from blame, self-recrimination, or disempowering fear. We help patients gain a broader understanding of cancer and the healing process, develop self-compassion, and create a practical action plan. In this way, patients develop a sense of regaining control and being in charge of their life and health. And that sense of control is a central element that helps in one's healing.

Whether you are active or passive, you have a major influence on your own healing. In a review of Bernard H. Fox's 2005 paper titled "The Role of Psychological Factors in Cancer Incidence and Prognosis" published in the journal *Oncology*, respected psychiatrist and cancer researcher Dr. David Spiegel wrote:

> Medicine has focused so much on attacking the tumor that it has tended to ignore the body coping with the tumor and the social and psychological variables that influence the somatic response to tumor invasion.
>
> Biologic treatments that produce only marginal increases in survival are widely employed despite considerable risks and side effects. Many psychosocial practices such as support groups, mind-body practices, and simple relaxation that are clearly helpful emotionally and carry with them very little in the way of risks, side effects, or expense are far less widely employed.

When we engage in creating our own health and healing from the broader integrative perspective, we become active and inspired participants in optimally supporting our mind, body, spirit, and immune system. Reclaiming a sense of control over our own life and health is a vitally important foundation for the healing process. By doing so, our immune system is enhanced, and we begin to actively work toward creating our own foundations for healing and recovery.

Autonomy and involvement in treatment decisions are important foundations of integrative medicine. All the complementary medical therapies we will discuss in this book are designed to support health and build immune function. And they are meant to do so in the least toxic and invasive manner.

My goal is to guide you in merging science with your inner wisdom to make choices that are optimal for you.

Yet for many breast cancer patients, the fact that many complementary therapies seem to lack the same scientific basis accorded surgery, radiation, or chemotherapy is a real problem. And it's true. While for some of these complementary therapies, substantial scientific evidence supports their use, for others, less research exists. I recognize that scientific evidence is a very helpful guide to choosing treatments. Evidence-informed care is valuable. But as Einstein said, "Not everything that counts can be counted, and not everything that can be counted counts." Trusting your own wisdom is also a very helpful guide to choosing treatments.

My goal is to guide you in merging science with your inner wisdom to make choices that are optimal for you.

The shift to the new model in breast health honors both the contributions and the limitations of orthodox cancer care. By removing or killing tumor cells, conventional cancer treatments can play a valuable role in reducing the tumor load with which the body has to deal. However, since many conventional cancer treatments also have negative effects on healthy cells, these same treatments are often associated with significant side effects that can substantially reduce both immune function and quality of life. Even worse, the long-term negative health consequences of these treatments often mean compromised health for the rest of one's life.

Complementary medical therapies function in an entirely different way. The goal of these therapies is to support the immune system and health, thus facilitating the body's healing abilities. They work together with the body to promote healing. Through this synergistic action, complementary therapies can support the body's health and improve quality of life. Plus, side effects from complementary treatment therapies are far less common.

No one who has participated in our cancer recovery program has ever developed a serious side effect from any of the complementary cancer therapies we have prescribed. More than two thousand years ago, Hippocrates, one of history's great physician healers, said, "Above all, do no harm," and "Honor the healing power of Nature." These principles guide the recommendations in this book.

The vast majority of participants in our program use both conventional and complementary modalities in an integrated way. We encourage participants to choose those therapies that feel right for them. This results in a truly individualized, integrated cancer care program. By providing information, choices, and options, personal autonomy is enhanced and healing is facilitated.

As you consider your own integrated breast cancer treatment program, please remember, conventional treatments do not address the underlying factors that predispose one to breast cancer development. Conventional breast cancer treatments address symptoms. The tumor model of breast cancer care considers the tumor the entire problem. The emerging model of breast cancer treatment recognizes the tumor as a physical indication of an underlying imbalance. And the condition of the body, mind, and spirit combined is the deciding factor in the required rebalance that leads to health and healing.

It's clear: The new model of breast care recognizes healthful nutrition and exercise are as important as any conventional cancer

The tumor model of breast cancer care considers the tumor the entire problem. The emerging model of breast cancer treatment recognizes the tumor as a physical indication of an underlying imbalance.

treatment. Plus emotional, social, and spiritual support add a deeper level of well-being than medicine alone can't offer.

The new model of breast care is grounded in helping your body's natural ability to get well and stay well. Gone is the total focus on the tumor as the problem. The new model focuses on the whole person, creating health and well-being physically, emotionally, and even spiritually. Of course, surgery, radiation, and chemotherapy may still play a role. But in the new model, it's not all about the treatment. It's about you. And that is very good news indeed.

2

Sources of Health and Healing

W HERE DO WE FIND HEALTH? How can we know healing? For the breast cancer patient, these are foundational questions. Thankfully, there is a hierarchy of answers.

The Will to Live

The will to live, a psychological force found within all of us, is your starting point. It can be easily understood as the *inner desire for survival*. The will to live is the most basic requirement for the breast cancer journey.

Like all creatures, human beings have a fierce instinct for survival. Sometimes the biology of breast cancer will dictate the course of events regardless of the patient's attitude and fighting spirit. These events are often beyond our control. But patients with positive attitudes are clearly better able to cope with disease-related problems. And many respond better to therapy.

O. Carl Simonton, MD, pointed out in his landmark book *Getting Well Again* that physicians often observe how two patients of similar ages, with the same diagnosis, sharing a similar degree of illness and virtually identical treatment programs, experience vastly different outcomes. One of the few apparent differences is that one patient was pessimistic and the other optimistic.

I often ask survivors to explain how they were able to transcend their health challenges.

We have known for more than two thousand years, from the writings of Plato and Galen, that there is a direct correlation between the mind, the body, and one's health. "The cure of many diseases is unknown to physicians," Plato concluded, "because they are ignorant of the whole. For the part can never be well unless the whole is well."

The new model of breast cancer care recognizes that the psychological and the physical elements of a body are not separate, isolated, and unrelated. Instead they are vitally linked elements of a total system. Health is increasingly recognized as a balance of many inputs, including physical and environmental factors, emotional and psychological states, nutritional habits, and exercise patterns.

Believe it. Your will to live plays a large role in your recovery. The mind's role in causing and curing disease has been endlessly debated. No studies have proven in a scientifically valid way that a person can control the course of his or her cancer with the mind alone. However, there are millions of individuals who attest to the power of positive attitudes and emotions. I am one of those individuals. I purposely cultivated and strengthened my will to live. You can too.

I often ask survivors to explain how they were able to transcend their health challenges. However diverse they are in ethnic or cultural background, age, educational level, or type of illness, they have all gone through a similar process of a psychological shift.

Virtually all consciously made a *decision to live*. After an initial period of feeling devastated, they simply decided to assess their new reality and live—however long that may be.

In my own case, when I decided to live, it meant that I wanted to enjoy life, to get more out of life, and to believe that my life was not over. It also meant that I was willing to do whatever was needed to make the very most of each day.

The threat of death often renews our appreciation of the importance of life, love, friendship, and all there is to enjoy. We open up to new possibilities and begin taking risks we didn't have the courage to take before. Many patients say that facing the uncertainties of living with an illness makes life more meaningful. The smallest pleasures are intensified, and much of the hypocrisy in life is eliminated. When pettiness, bitterness, and anger begin to dissipate, there is still a capacity for joy. I want that for you.

One patient wrote, "I love living, I love nature. Being outdoors, feeling the sun on my face and the wind blowing against my body, hearing birds sing, breathing in the spray of the ocean. I never lose hope that I may somehow be graced with a victory against this disease."

Quite understandably, many patients react to the diagnosis of breast cancer in the same way that people in primitive cultures reacted to a witch doctor's curse or spell; they see it as a death sentence. This phenomenon, known as bone pointing, results in a paralytic fear that causes the victim to simply withdraw from the world and await the inevitable end. In modern medical practice, a similar phenomenon may occur when, out of ignorance or superstition, a patient believes the diagnosis of cancer to be a death sentence. The good news is that the phenomenon of self-willed death is only effective if the person believes in the power of the curse. And we can change our beliefs.

Hope: The Force That Sets Your Course

Combining the will to live with hope creates health and healing.

Cicero, the Roman statesman, is credited with the phrase "While there is life, there is hope." I believe those words have greater power in reverse: "While there is hope, there is life." Hope comes first; life follows. Hope is the force that sets your course, inspiring the will to live and healing on every level.

The dictionary defines hope as a feeling that what is wanted can be had, that events will turn out for the best. That is not strong enough. Hope can best be defined as deeply confident expectation. It is a force; a mental, emotional, and spiritual power; a strength you possess. Hope gives power to life to continue, expand, reach out, and go on. Hope is the miracle medicine of the mind. It inspires the will to live. Hope is the patient's greatest ally.

I ask that you stop to consider the importance of hope in your breast cancer journey. Please allow me to gently ask you three questions:

Do you carry a vision of yourself as struggling or victorious?

Do you believe disease or health is in your future?

Do you live most of each day filled with helplessness or hopefulness?

How you envision yourself and perceive your circumstances has a great deal to do with your actual life experience. It's true in all areas of life—our relationships, our work, and especially our health.

One essential key to unlocking health is to carry a vision of hope. Hope revives ideals, renews dreams, and revitalizes visions. Hope scales the peak, wrestles with the impossible, and achieves the highest aim. Carry this truth deep in your heart: as long as you have hope, you are not helpless and no situation is hopeless.

A powerful act in creating health and healing is to choose the words you speak. Our words may sometimes spring forth without thought. But we have a choice. Words matter. Words are powerful. They can create either good or bad, health or illness. We can stop speaking about our problems and start speaking of our healing. The more we speak of solutions, as if they already exist, the less powerful our problems become. I ask that from this moment forward, you begin to speak only of health and of healing. When you do, you plant the seeds to help create that reality.

A surgeon once admonished me, "You're spreading false hope." My response was "I believe there is no such thing as false hope. I believe there is only reasonable hope." There is, however, a great deal of false hopelessness. In medicine, that often takes shape in words like "There's nothing more we can do." Or "You have only months to live." Don't believe them.

Your mind is similar to this computer at which I am working. Your mind stores virtually every thought and impression you've ever had. Just now I can recall the happy thoughts of my first bicycle. That was decades ago. Your mind also stores a lot of garbage—negative input that we are inundated with every day. And a great deal of that garbage is all about what's wrong, what's hopeless in our lives. Reject the garbage. Refuse to dwell on anything that is hopeless. See yourself smiling, vital, and fully alive. Fill your mind with visions of health, happiness, and peace.

Clearly, it is unrealistic to pretend that nothing bad ever happens to us. Bad things do happen to good people. Breast cancer is one of those bad things. Pretending otherwise is not the answer. Nor is playing word games to make ourselves sound psychologically strong or spiritually pure. When bad things happen, admit it. Acknowledge the breast cancer, but keep your thoughts focused on the most hopeful outcome.

We simply must take personal responsibility for our thoughts and words. As long as we keep making excuses and blaming our family tree, our doctor, or even God, we will never be truly well, because excuses and blame give away our personal power. As a result, we will never be filled with the overcoming power of hope.

I say this lovingly: It's not the diagnosis of breast cancer that has you struggling and depressed. No. It's your thoughts about your diagnosis and circumstances that keep you down.

Know this: we can control our thoughts and our words. And through that control, we can influence, to a very large extent, our health and our life. I ask you to exercise that control.

We can control our thoughts and our words. And through that control, we can influence, to a very large extent, our health and our life. I ask you to exercise that control.

A group of us were game fishing in the Atlantic Ocean. I had no idea which direction land was. So I asked our captain, "How do you know the way back?" He pointed to a large built-in compass just above the wheel. "From here," he said. "Just keep that compass on north." So, too, in your journey through breast cancer. If you want to know and experience the best of health and healing, set your compass on true north—set it on hope.

In front of the Cancer Recovery Group's offices is a five-thousand-pound slab of Vermont granite. I've had the Rules of Survivorship inscribed on it. Here they are:

Rule 1: There is always hope.

Rule 2: If someone says there is no hope, reread rule 1.

Believe it. There is always hope. Let that sink deep into your mind and spirit. Hope is the force that sets your course. Follow the rules. Set your compass on hope. Keep your mind filled with victory! It is one of the great sources of health and healing.

Spiritual Connection: Inner Guidance

Healing is a very personal journey, unique in its path for each of us. At our deepest intuitive levels, many of us know the most important things we need to do to get well and stay well. However, millions of us have forgotten how to listen to and trust our intuitive inner wisdom. Connecting with your own sense of what it means to be spiritual is an essential step to defining your path to wellness.

Breast cancer is a call to listen to your Self—your Inner Healer, your deeper wisdom. Caught up in life's busyness, we often forget how to relax the mind and quiet the spirit. But it is only when we can be at peace and surrender to our deeper wisdom that we can receive the inner guidance so essential to healing.

I ask you, beginning today, to quiet your mind long enough to discover your own healing pathway. What you will find is both surprising and exciting. Research in psychospiritual reality confirms what healers and spiritual teachers have known for centuries—at the level of Self, we are far more aware and knowledgeable than at the level of our conscious mind.

Prayer is one method of rediscovering our Self. For many people, this spiritual journey may be expressed through a religious framework. And for others, spirituality is expressed through a connection with Nature or a similar quest. The common thread is to connect with our deepest authentic Self. And for the skeptics, we now even have early research to show that this quest can activate the immune system, promote healing, and increase possibilities for recovery.

In our work, we have found the spiritual journey to healing can be reliably and predictably started with three practices—forgiveness, gratitude, and unconditional love.

Forgiveness is our letting go of hurts and grievances. To be clear, it is our offering of forgiveness to others, not our receipt of forgiveness from others, which makes the difference. And most of us know at a deep level the thoughts of recrimination and remorse to which we cling. It was only after I forgave my father that I was able to reclaim health and receive the gift of healing. Release. Let go. Forgive. It opens the door to the Self.

Gratitude is a state of living and being consciously aware of and appreciative of the countless blessings and kindnesses we receive every moment. So very often on the cancer journey, our sense of gratitude can be momentarily clouded by helplessness, doubt, and despair. When we observe and affirm the good things in life, we see them expand and open the door to the hidden Self.

Unconditional loving—I like the word *loving* rather than the word *love*, since it better communicates the action required to actualize love—is the essential practice of spiritual connection. Unconditional loving is another and higher state of Self. It comprises giving, creative flow, and harmony. It's the acceptance of the human condition as perfectly imperfect. And it is a choice to love without any qualifications; no ifs are allowed.

> *Release. Let go. Forgive. It opens the door to the Self.*

Forgiveness, gratitude, and unconditional loving. They are the gateway to your Self, to spiritual connection and inner guidance—one of the most powerful sources of health and healing. We will have more to say on these in the 50 Essential Things You Can Do.

Relationships: Emotional Intelligence and Support

One of the great wellsprings of healing is an intimate group of supportive friends. When combined with a keen understanding of our emotional makeup, the environment for healing is optimized.

We are in the realm of our feelings. Fear, anger, and guilt. Happiness, contentment, and love. They are all part of the human experience. Emotions are especially vivid when we are dealing with a life-threatening illness. In the breast cancer experience, we cannot expect to prevent negative emotions altogether, nor should we expect to experience positive feelings every moment.

But what we can do is acknowledge our feelings and refuse to get stuck in the negative ones. That often takes the help of one or more true friends.

You and I have the power to choose our emotions. Recall the concept that body, mind, and spirit all work together. Emotions are clearly part of that mix. When we recognize that our every thought, word, and behavior affects our greater health and well-being, we have begun to learn the language of emotions.

Emotions are very often misunderstood. In most cultures, emotions are either repressed or acted out in unhealthy or uncontrolled ways. Anger kills—literally and figuratively. Love heals. And once we learn to recognize an emotion like joy, we can utilize this vital resource to move toward wholeness and more vibrant health on our cancer journey.

Please understand that your emotions actually do manifest in your physical body and yield physical sensations. Take anxiety as an example. You may be anxious over an upcoming series of medical tests. Before long, you notice you have an upset stomach. Your first response might be to avoid or deny the connection. But if you stop and become aware of the sequence of thoughts and emotions, you can begin to develop a felt sense of these emotions and their link to your body. As a result, you can respond in a more intelligent way.

With practice, we can become skilled at observing our emotions. And once we can put words to the emotions—"That's fear I am feeling," for example—we tend to no longer fight the emotion.

Instead, we can allow the emotion to work through without repression or strong reaction.

As a result, we begin to experience more ease, more joy, and more spontaneity in our lives. We are now able to claim a more honest relationship with ourselves, and our relationships with others also become more authentic.

Research in the field of psychoneuroimmunology attests to the central role emotions play in the healing process. Landmark studies have demonstrated that simply meeting with others once a week to connect emotionally and to provide mutual support strengthens one's sense of well-being and significantly improves the chance of recovery from life-threatening illness.

UCLA cancer researcher Dr. Fawzy Fawzy found that cancer patients randomly assigned to participate in a weekly support group for a six-week period after diagnosis were much more likely to be alive five years later than those who were not in a group.

In San Francisco, Dr. David Spiegel found that women with metastatic breast cancer who attended a weekly support meeting lived, on average, twice as long as those who did not. Patients were encouraged to express their feelings about the illness and its effect on their lives. Spiegel found that the emotional repression and social isolation so often found among breast cancer patients was countered by participation in these groups. Importantly, he also noted that group members encouraged one another to be more assertive with their doctors.

In Arizona, Dr. Karen Weihs demonstrated that for women diagnosed with breast cancer, a large group of supportive friends and relatives is associated with a 60 percent reduction in recurrence and death compared to women with breast cancer who were socially isolated.

> *Share with these people how important they are in your life. And recognize that the contribution made by their support is as important as any breast cancer therapy.*

It's clear. Emotional connection with oneself and one's family and friends plays a pivotal role in the healing process. As you spend time with those you love, do not simply rehearse the problems of breast cancer. Instead, share with these people how important they are in your life. And recognize that the contribution made by their support is as important as any breast cancer therapy.

Mind-Body: Visualizing the Desired Outcome

As you already know, I am asking you to understand the incredible healing potential you possess. For many people, the body's ability to heal remains a greatly underutilized resource. In large part it is because we have forgotten how to listen to the healing messages our body gives us. If we just take the time to reconnect with our healing wisdom, we can tap in to the resources of emotion, memory, and imagery. Then we find an awakened sense of wholeness, and we can activate this mind-body connection to support our immune system and promote healing.

What we think and feel directly impacts our health. Research has demonstrated that mind power can translate to muscle power. In a fascinating study, medical researchers explained the health benefits of the physical activity involved with the work of hospital cleaning staff. Once understood, the employees lost body fat, decreased their blood pressure, and increased their lean muscle mass. Their activity levels did not change. The only difference was what they were told about their work. Researchers concluded that increased awareness accounted for the health gains.

Some people dismiss this as the placebo effect, the well-documented and sustained outcomes in response to treatment with a sugar pill versus actual medication. But even placebo effects should not be dismissed—if and when we believe in a treatment, that belief itself nurtures health. Our mind is a powerful tool to assist healing.

The mind can be quickly employed in the quest for healing. Simply by visualizing thoughts, images, and pictures of healing through use of the imagination, our body's defense mechanisms can respond. Cortisol levels that inhibit maximum immune function drop. Endorphin levels rise, indicating increased immune activity.

In my own case, I employed the phrase "I am cancer free, a picture of health." Concurrently I would imagine myself vital and alive, arms outstretched overhead, reaching to the clear blue skies, with a big smile on my face.

I ask you to try something similar. Or you may wish to seek guidance from someone else or by listening to a recording. The point is the mind-body connection can be triggered through visualization, guided imagery, and affirmation.

Although these techniques and modalities enhance the mind-body connection, simply listening to and honoring what your body is telling you to do is a good start. For example, fatigue is the single most common symptom in people with cancer. From the perspective of integrated cancer care, fatigue is our body's way of telling us to rest and to take time for self-care. Listen to what your body is telling you. Feel your energy level. And adjust your activity levels accordingly.

As we quiet our mind and deepen the intimate connection with our body, we can hear what our body is telling us. I am asking you to notice your mind, to listen to and nurture your body's healing wisdom. It is a powerful source of health.

You will find examples of visualization exercises in Appendix 5: "Meditation and Visualization."

Physical Exercise: The Five-Hour Standard

"I'm too tired."

"It's no fun."

"I don't have the time."

"My legs look ugly in gym shorts."

"The weather's bad."

You've heard them. I've used them. They are excuses people use when they don't want to exercise. But even the very best of integrated cancer care will not be maximized without regular exercise. Think of it as a mandatory requirement.

In 2005, the *Journal of the American Medical Association* published a study on physical activity and survival after a breast cancer diagnosis. The study found that exercising just one hour per week could lower the risk of recurrence by approximately 20 percent. And the risk of recurrence was reduced by 50 percent when the exercise time was increased to three to five hours per week.

The benefits of exercise before, during, and after cancer treatment are now appearing frequently in medical research. When we started our work more than a quarter century ago, Cancer Recovery Group was the first organization to document the link between exercise and recovery. At that time, we did not clearly understand the answers to the questions, How much exercise? and What type? Today, the answers are much clearer. On the whole, you and I need to make daily exercise a part of our lives.

Cancer and its treatments cause significant changes in the body, including fatigue, muscle weakness, and loss of flexibility that can make normal daily activities challenging. Movement counters these changes and becomes a key aspect of recovery and healing. Something as simple as gentle-range-of-motion exercise following breast surgery enhances energy, increases flexibility, improves mood, and often produces an overall feeling of greater well-being.

Mild exercise such as a brisk walk, housecleaning, and gardening improves quality of life, sleep, and appetite. Moderate exercise also reduces the risks of heart disease, high blood pressure, diabetes, osteoporosis, anxiety, and depression. As noted, exercise reduces the risk of breast cancer recurrence by naturally suppressing estrogen production in menstruating women. Of course it follows that cumulative lifetime exposure to estrogen is also reduced.

At our affiliate, Breast Cancer Charities of America, we have helped set the aerobic standard for minimum exercise at twenty to forty minutes three to five times per week. In 2006, a study found this level to be safe for cancer patients receiving chemotherapy. From our survivor interviews, we know that only 30 percent of breast cancer patients meet that standard. I am asking you to join that select group of women. And I am further encouraging you to be at the high end of the standard.

You owe it to yourself to schedule a walk each and every day. Or perhaps you prefer gentle yoga or Qigong, both of which combine relaxation and exercise. I ask you to exercise out of doors whenever possible. The fresh air and the exposure to sunlight are sources of health on their own.

The physiology of regular exercise facilitates the flow of lymphatic fluid. I liken our lymph system to a series of hydraulic chambers. The motions of moderate exercise help keep these fluids moving from chamber to chamber. And with that flow, our immune system more effectively eliminates toxins, bacteria, and abnormal cells. Unlike the circulatory system, which relies on the heart to pump blood, the lymphatic system has no pump. Instead, lymph function relies on the contraction of our muscles during our activities of daily living to move lymphatic fluid through the system.

Moderate exercise also helps minimize lymphedema in breast cancer patients. This is the often painful fluid buildup many patients experience postsurgery and especially following removal of lymph nodes. Researchers examined the association between lymphedema and exercise and found that upper-body weight training did not increase the risk of lymphedema; it helped. It is reasonable to conclude that breast cancer patients can and should engage in moderate upper-body resistance training.

Take these exercise guidelines very seriously. The costs of failing to exercise are simply too great. Start slow. Find the right routine. Do something every day—no excuses. Okay, end of lecture.

To further support maximum lymph function, drink at least eight glasses of water per day. This helps provide the needed hydration that optimizes lymphatic volume and fluid.

As much as I strive to make the message of this book gentle, personal, and filled with hope, I now need to deliver a short but loving lecture: Take these exercise guidelines very seriously. The costs of failing to exercise are simply too great. Start slow. Find the right routine. Do something every day—no excuses. Okay, end of lecture.

Just do it! Join me in making daily exercise a central part of your life. Soon it will become more than a requirement; it will become a pleasure. And then you will know you are truly on the path to health and healing.

Nutrition: The Most Healthful Choice

"Eat a plant." If you are dealing with breast cancer, that is the one best and most distilled nugget of nutritional advice I can possibly convey to you. Yes, "eat a plant."

The breast cancer patient's guide to nutrition is simple and easily implemented. The best foods are predominantly fresh and organically grown fruits, vegetables, whole grains, and legumes. We also favor beans, nuts, and seeds. Choose fish, some soy and soy alternatives, and egg whites in their natural form. It is preferable if the source of these foods is local.

What you are seeking are the wholesome foods that nature provides. This means to avoid processed foods, refined foods, and those that contain toxic chemicals and additives. It also means we spend a great deal of our time shopping for food in the produce section of our market.

Cancer remains much less prevalent in cultures that continue to eat the unrefined foods of our ancestors. And while modern technology has enabled us to mass-produce foods for high yields, long shelf life, and maximum profits, it is clear that nutritional values have been compromised in the process. Factory farming has changed the health integrity of our food. As a result, most people are missing essential nutrients that were commonplace in previous generations.

Since you or a loved one is dealing with breast cancer, now is the time to launch an extreme nutritional makeover. It starts by eating actual food—that means quality, real, natural food. If it is boxed or bottled or canned or packaged, be skeptical. A nutrition makeover means asking questions as you shop. How fresh are these ingredients? Where was it grown? Is it local? Is it organic? What does this label tell me? Does this contain genetically modified ingredients? And more.

I am not asking you to go on a diet. I am asking you to change and improve your lifestyle. If you think you are going on a diet, chances are that you'll go off that diet. Sooner or later, for most people, being on a diet—any diet—is simply not sustainable. The word *diet* itself conjures up images of deprivation and restrictions. Nobody wants to be deprived and restricted.

In contrast, I am asking you to adopt high-nutrition as a wonderful way of life. There is no diet to get on or get off. The breast cancer recovery nutrition program gives you maximum choices that taste good. It is satisfying and nutritious. And it fights cancer.

In his book *Food Rules*, Michael Pollan brilliantly distills the nutrition discussion into seven words. He says, "Eat food. Not too much. Mostly plants."

Eat food: Not the highly processed, nutritionally void, prepackaged foods so common in most grocery stores. Eat real-life, high-quality food. Pollan gives powerful advice when he says, "It's not food if it arrived through the window of your car." I love it!

> *The word* diet *itself conjures up images of deprivation and restrictions. Nobody wants to be deprived and restricted.*

Not too much: This is portion control. And unless you are in the stages of breast cancer where you simply cannot maintain weight, the Scottish guideline "A little with quiet is the only diet" serves you well. Yet the good thing about a plant-based program is that you can eat more—up to ten servings a day of fresh vegetables and fruit.

Mostly plants: Not exclusively plants, but predominantly plants—whole foods that are organically grown and filled with the thousands of natural phytonutrients that help create health and healing.

While there are few Thou Shalt Nots in the breast cancer recovery nutrition program, there is one: avoid refined sugar. White sugar and other forms of refined sugar are to be avoided altogether. This includes raw sugar, brown sugar, evaporated cane sugar, and corn syrup. This also means avoiding processed foods that contain these sugars. And it extends to foods that contain fructose, glucose, and dextrose. In addition, avoid all artificial or chemical sweeteners such as sorbitol, xylitol, and mannitol.

I have previously written about cancer feeding on sugar. I stand by that analysis. Avoid refined sugar. (I discuss this more in "#21 Adopt This Nutritional Strategy" in chapter 7.)

When you find it necessary to sweeten foods or drinks, use stevia, a natural herb that can be used freely. This sweetener is now widely available in liquid, powder, or tablet form. Just ask at your local market. If you simply must find other sugar alternatives, use small amounts of natural sweeteners such as raw or unpasteurized honey, real maple syrup, whole unrefined sugar, or blackstrap molasses.

Finally, add generous amounts of health-enhancing superfoods. They are comprised of plants that have extraordinary anticancer effects. These include various kinds of cabbage, broccoli, garlic, several kinds of mushrooms, green tea, turmeric, raspberries, blueberries, strawberries, certain nuts, several herbs and spices, and even dark chocolate—although in smaller amounts. Healthful choices are explored in detail in the Food as Medicine appendixes.

Know this: healthful food is one of the primary sources of health and healing. What you eat is central to your recovery from breast cancer. Food's influence is considerable—every day, three times a day—either speeding up or slowing down cancer growth. Just like we spoke of exercise, I urge you to take this nutritional guidance very seriously. Eating unhealthfully is simply too big a risk if you wish to recover from breast cancer.

Where do we find health? How can we know healing? It's right before us. And many breast cancer patients, in the rush to find a conventional or complementary treatment, overlook the true sources that make for health and healing. The elements we have explored here are essential aspects of self-care and of health. Without these strong foundations, even the most exotic breast cancer treatments will crumble. We simply must do more than treat the illness. We must create wellness.

3

Medicine: Consider the Whole

FOR MOST WOMEN, MEDICINE TENDS to be the first and only consideration in the breast cancer journey. That is unfortunate but true. Given this is the case, it is helpful to possess an understanding of the typical processes involved in the tumor model of breast cancer care.

Diagnosis: What to Expect

A series of predictable events begins when a suspicious lump needs to be definitively diagnosed. You should expect, or may have already experienced, something similar to the following from your primary care physician:

1. A mammogram.

2. A review of your health history that led up to the mammogram.

3. An explanation of the properties that might differentiate a malignant lump from a benign lump.

4. A review of the results of the mammogram focusing on the perceived type of lump and whether or not additional lesions were detected in either breast.

5. A recommendation and review on methods that may need to be implemented to confirm if the suspect lump is malignant. These recommendations may include:

a. Ultrasound

Ultrasounds are used to distinguish cysts from solid tumors. This tool uses high-frequency sound waves that are pulsed through the breast tissue. When the sound waves meet a solid obstacle, like a tumor, they bounce back. When they encounter fluid or normal tissue, they pass through the breast. Ultrasounds are best at examining one lump or area of concern that has already been detected by physical exam or mammography. They are not effective as a stand-alone breast screening method. Ultrasounds are harmless and do not expose you to radiation.

Cancers and fibroadenomas are solid, while cysts are hollow and filled with fluid. If the ultrasound demonstrates that the lump is filled with fluid, a biopsy is not necessary. If it shows that the mass is solid, then a biopsy must be carried out to determine whether it is a fibroadenoma or cancer.

The ultrasound can be carried out before a mammogram when a cyst is suspected. If it is a cyst, there is no need for a mammogram, and you are spared radiation exposure.

b. Magnetic Resonance Imaging (MRI)

MRIs are most useful in imaging early breast cancers, particularly in women with genetic susceptibility who require annual screening for breast cancer before the age of forty. This is the time of life when mammography is least accurate due to increased breast density. In these women, MRIs are more accurate than mammography, ultrasound, and clinical breast exams.

MRIs do not expose women to radiation but rather use a huge magnet to image tissues after a contrast dye is injected intravenously. The dye is absorbed more easily by cancer cells than by normal tissue or benign lesions. The disadvantages of MRIs are their expense, a high level of false positive test results, and the need for several doctors and technicians trained in interpreting breast MRIs.

c. Fine Needle Aspiration

Fine needle aspiration is easy to perform, relatively pain-less, and can be carried out in a doctor's office. A needle is inserted into the tumor, and fluid is removed. If clear fluid is removed and the tumor dissolves, it was a simple cyst. If the fluid is bloody, cancer with a cystic component may exist. The fluid is then sent to the pathology lab for analysis.

If no fluid is obtained, a biopsy must be performed. Fine needle aspiration is the least invasive, fastest, and most inexpensive way to diagnose breast cancer, provided the physician is skilled in the technique. A growing number of doctors believe that fine needle aspiration should be per-formed on all palpable breast masses. A diagnosis is estab-lished with this technique 90 percent of the time.

d. Biopsy

A biopsy will confirm or negate the presence of cancer if the above tests have not been definitive. A sample of tissue is taken in one of two ways and then analyzed.

The first method is called open surgical biopsy and is ideally performed as a lumpectomy. This means to treat a suspicious lump as though the diagnosis of cancer had already been made. This reduces the need for a second sur-gery should the first demonstrate breast cancer. The method also reduces scarring. The whole mass is removed along with a margin of normal tissue so that a pathologist can be sure that all the edges of the cancer have been taken out and nothing remains.

The second method is called a core biopsy. For a large palpable mass, one to six slender cores of tissue are taken from different sites within it. It is most accurate for larger lesions and is much less invasive than an open surgical biopsy.

Choices of these diagnostic procedures depend on the technol-ogy that is available in your geographical area as well as the prevail-ing local medical customs. In addition, the experience of the family physician and the diagnostician will also influence the recommendations. One hopes the recommendations align with best practice and best outcome guidelines.

Once one or more of these procedures are completed, you are hopefully given a clean bill of health. If not, you then experience one of the most difficult parts of the breast cancer journey, waiting for lab reports. In my experience, more "awfulizing"—taking thoughts to their worst possible conclusion—takes place during the wait for test results than at any other time in the cancer journey. I'll have more to say about how to control awfulizing in "#1 Focus" in chapter 7, "The 50 Essential Things You Can Do."

Information: Seeing Through the Haze

At this point in the process, you no doubt have researched information on breast cancer. If you have access to the Internet, the information can be overwhelming. And if you visit some of the government sites, the technical nature of the information is often confusing.

It is very helpful to have a practical working knowledge of breast cancer and its physiology. The next section will discuss this subject in a nontechnical way with the hope that you will gain an understanding of what it is that you, or the loved one you support, are dealing with.

The Look and Feel of Breast Cancer

Most often, breast cancer is felt as a hard, irregular-shaped, non-tender lump. The size of the lump varies, but hopefully the lump in question is small. The lump does not float throughout the breast but often feels as though it is attached to underlying tissue.

There also may be breast redness, swelling, and even the feel of warmth. A puckering of the skin near the lump site is common. The shape and contour of the breast may undergo noticeable changes. With inflammatory breast cancer, there may even be a vague orange-peel look characterized by a thick, pitted appearance of the breast's skin. In more advanced diagnoses, bloody nipple discharge, an inverted nipple, and changes in nipple size may occur. And at some point, swollen lymph nodes in the armpit may appear.

Cancer Cells and Tumors

Cancer cells are often present ten years before a mass is finally detectable, having grown to a size one centimeter in diameter and consisting of one billion cells. The time required for one cell to divide into two cells is called doubling time, and the rate varies between about 21 and 188 days, depending on breast cancer type and age. Aggressive cancers have a faster doubling time.

Given a healthy lifestyle, a cell normally has the capacity to repair itself. Cells from our immune system also constantly survey the body, on guard for precancerous cells. When normal cell repair is unable to keep with them, though, the cancerous cells duplicate the damage as they divide and reproduce themselves. This is the start of a malignant condition. Several hormones, including excess estrogen and insulin, contribute to the faster multiplication of breast cells and accelerate the rate at which damaged cells form a tumor, though they may not have caused the original genetic defect.

When the clump of aberrant cells spreads out from the tissue of origin to the surrounding area, it is classified as invasive cancer. Nutritional substances, such as vitamin D, all the carotenoids, zinc, iodine, and flaxseed oil, help protect the lining of the breast ducts and lobules to be more resistant to invasion by cancer cells. Many foods and nutrients, such as garlic, fish oil, tomatoes, red berries, beans, and bran help to slow this growth phase.

If the tumor reaches a critical size of about two millimeters, about the thickness of a dime, it sends out chemical signals to recruit blood vessels. When blood vessels form to bring it nutrients, the tumor grows much faster. Environmental estrogens may help it to do this. Green tea, turmeric, and zinc help prevent the formation of this blood supply, known as angiogenesis, as well as stall the growth phase.

The essential concept to grasp is that breast cancer begins with changes in the DNA of the cell. This action is initiated by a variety of causative agents, including chemicals, radicals, toxic metals, electromagnetic fields, genetic defects, drugs, viruses, and stress. A healthy lifestyle is the number one deterrent to the onset of breast cancer. Once again, as we create health, we transcend disease.

A healthy lifestyle is the number one deterrent to the onset of breast cancer. Once again, as we create health, we transcend disease.

Metastasis

Single cancer cells can separate from the original tumor and travel through the blood or lymphatic vessels to the rest of the body. They can migrate to the liver, lungs, bone marrow, or brain and multiply to form another tumor, or metastasis, of the original deranged breast cell.

The body tries to put a halt to this process by attacking breast cancer cells in the lymph nodes and sending out white blood cells to patrol the blood, seeking and destroying any wandering cancer cells. Melatonin levels increase in an attempt to curtail the cancerous process. Note that melatonin is produced naturally through sun exposure. And vitamin D acts as an inhibitor of metastasis.

Unlike normal cells, cancer cells lose the signal to die after they reproduce. They are on a narcissistic mission of self-perpetuation at the expense of their host. Over time, they can interfere with processes essential to life. Many natural substances can be used to inhibit metastases. For more information, see the nutritional guidelines in the 50 Essential Things You Can Do.

Types of Breast Cancer

There are approximately thirty types of breast cancer that include a series of grades and stages indicating severity and complexity. But for our purposes, we can divide breast cancer into two main categories, lobular and ductal. Most breast cancers are ductal.

The term *carcinoma in situ* is used for the early stage of cancer, when it is limited to the immediate area where it began. Specifically in breast cancer, *in situ* means that the cancer remains confined to the ducts or lobules. It has not invaded surrounding tissues in the breast, nor has it spread to other organs in the body. If the cancer moves from the site of origin, it is called invasive.

Most breast cancers begin in glandular tissue, such as the ducts or lobules of the breast. They are called adenocarcinomas, *adeno* meaning "related to a gland." About 86 percent of breast cancers start in the ducts, while 12 percent originate in the lobules at the end of the ducts.

Ductal Carcinoma in Situ (DCIS)

Ductal carcinoma in situ, also known as intraductal carcinoma, or DCIS, is the most common type of noninvasive breast cancer. *Noninvasive* means that the cancer cells are inside the ducts but have not spread through the walls of the ducts into the surrounding breast tissue. Approximately 25 percent of all new breast cancer patients are found to have DCIS.

One of the great mysteries about breast cancer is what to make of DCIS. These tumors are so small they cannot be felt. Studies show that most stay in the milk ducts, where they originate, never spreading to the rest of the breast where they can become lethal. The problem is that doctors cannot tell the dangerous DCIS tumors from the harmless ones, so they treat all such tumors as if they are dangerous.

There are a growing number of breast cancer experts who debate whether DCIS should actually be classified as breast cancer. Predictably, the discussion over this point is heated. And the prevailing conventional wisdom is "DCIS is breast cancer. Get it out." This leads to massive overtreatment. I believe the evidence is overwhelming that DCIS is reversible through lifestyle choices. Much of this book expands on this view.

Lobular Carcinoma in Situ (LCIS)

Although it is not a true cancer, Lobular Carcinoma in Situ, or LCIS, also called lobular neoplasia, is sometimes classified as a type of noninvasive breast cancer. It is uncommon, occurring in about 2 percent of all breast biopsies. The atypical cells begin in the otherwise hollow milk-producing glands and can fill them up. They do not penetrate through the wall of the lobules. Usually LCIS does not become an invasive cancer. But women with this condition do have an increased risk of developing cancer in either breast within thirty years. If a cancer does occur, it isn't necessarily confined to where the original LCIS was discovered, but it can arise in any place in either breast. The point is, whatever is causing LCIS also puts these women at risk for future cancer.

Infiltrating Ductal Carcinoma (IDC)

Infiltrating Ductal Carcinoma, also called Invasive Ductal Carcinoma, or IDC, starts in a milk duct of the breast, breaks through the wall of the duct, and invades the fatty tissue of the breast. It usually feels like a hard, firm lump or an irregularly shaped mass of varying density and mobility, with fibrous extensions into the surrounding breast tissue that can create a crab-like appearance. The scar tissue that forms around ductal cancer cells creates the feeling of hardness.

There is about a 15 percent chance of this cancer occurring in the other breast. Invasive ductal carcinoma may metastasize, or spread to other parts of the body, such as the liver, brain, bones, or lungs, through the lymphatic system and bloodstream.

Medullary Carcinoma

Medullary Carcinoma is a special type of infiltrating breast cancer that has a rather well-defined, distinct boundary between tumor tissue and normal tissue. It has some other special features, including the large size of the cancer cells and the presence of immune system cells at the edges of the tumor. Medullary carcinoma accounts for about 5 percent of breast cancers. Because of its less aggressive nature, medullary carcinoma rarely mestastasizes to distant sites.

Tubular Carcinoma

Tubular carcinomas are a special type of infiltrating breast carcinoma in which the cancer cells look like small tubes. They account for less than 2 percent of all breast cancers and are usually less aggressive than other infiltrating ductal or lobular carcinomas.

Infiltrating Lobular Carcinoma (ILC)

Infiltrating lobular carcinoma, or Invasive Lobular Carcinoma or ILC, starts in the milk-producing glands, or lobules. This type of cancer can also spread to other parts of the body. About 10 percent of invasive cancers are ILCs. Invasive lobular carcinoma may be harder to detect by mammography than invasive ductal carcinoma.

Inflammatory Breast Cancer

Inflammatory breast cancer is invasive and rare, accounting for about 1 percent of all breast cancers. It makes the skin of the breast look red and feel warm and gives the skin a thick, pitted appearance. These changes are not caused by inflammation or infection but by cancer cells blocking lymph vessels or channels.

Paget's Disease

Paget's disease begins in the breast ducts and spreads to the nipple and then to the areola, the dark circle around the nipple. It is rare, accounting for only 1 to 5 percent of all cases of breast cancer. The skin of the nipple and areola often appears crusted, scaly, and red, with areas of bleeding, ulceration, and oozing, similar to eczema. Symptoms may also include burning or itching of the skin around the nipple. Paget's disease may be associated with in situ (noninvasive) or with invasive breast cancer. About half the time, a painless mass can be felt underneath the reddened area, which is usually indicative of invasive cancer. If no lump can be felt in the breast tissue, and the biopsy shows DCIS but no invasive cancer, the prognosis is excellent.

Phyllodes Tumor

A phyllodes tumor is a very rare type of breast cancer that develops in the stroma (connective tissue) of the breast, in contrast to carcinomas, which begin in the ducts or lobules. Phyllodes tumors are usually benign but on rare occasions may be malignant.

Benign phyllodes tumors are treated by removing the mass and a narrow margin of breast tissue. A malignant phyllodes tumor is treated by taking it out along with a wider margin of normal tissue, or by mastectomy. These cancers do not respond to hormonal therapies and are not as likely to respond to chemotherapy or radiation therapy. In the past, both benign and malignant phyllodes tumors were referred to as cystosarcoma phyllodes.

Stages of Breast Cancer

The stages of breast cancer are ranked to reflect the severity of the disease or the threat to life. They are labeled Stage 0, I, II, III, or IV.

Stage 0: Stage 0 is carcinoma in situ, which 75 to 80 percent of the time does not progress to invasive cancer.

Stage I: Stage I is when the tumor is smaller than two centimeters and there is no lymph node involvement.

Stage II: Stage II occurs when the tumor is smaller than two centimeters with lymph node involvement, or when the tumor is between two and five centimeters with positive or negative lymph nodes, or when it is larger than five centimeters with no lymph node involvement.

Stage III: Stage III is when the tumor is larger than five centimeters with positive lymph nodes, possible skin involvement, and/or when the tumor is fixed to the chest wall.

Stage IV: Stage IV occurs when the cancer has metastasized to a distant site or the diagnosis is inflammatory carcinoma.

Conventional Breast Cancer Treatments

It is also helpful to have a brief overview of the main types of breast cancer treatments. This section will give you that information. While conventional treatments do not equate with cure, they do provide help for many patients. For those readers who wish more detailed information, I recommend you visit *www.mayoclinic.com/health/breast-cancer/DS00328*.

Surgery

Surgery is usually the first treatment response to a breast cancer diagnosis.

Decisions about surgery depend on many factors. With your doctor, you will determine the kind of surgery that's most appropriate based on the stage of the cancer, the expression of the cancer, and what is acceptable to you in terms of your long-term peace of mind.

Your discussion with your surgeon will typically include an understanding of lumpectomy versus mastectomy. Lumpectomy, also known as breast-conserving surgery, is the removal of only the tumor and a small amount of surrounding tissue. Mastectomy is the removal of all of the breast tissue. Although no longer as common, mastectomy may include removing the muscles under the breast.

Lymph node removal, or axillary lymph node dissection, may take place during lumpectomy and mastectomy if the biopsy shows that breast cancer has spread outside the milk duct. Many patients qualify for the less-invasive sentinel lymph node dissection.

Breast reconstruction is the rebuilding of the breast after mastectomy and sometimes lumpectomy. Reconstruction can take place at the same time as cancer surgery. Or it may be done months or even years later. Some women decide not to have reconstruction and opt for a prosthesis instead.

Prophylactic mastectomy is preventive removal of the breast to lower the risk of breast cancer in high-risk people.

Prophylactic ovary removal is a preventive surgery that lowers the amount of estrogen in the body, making it harder for estrogen to stimulate the development of breast cancer.

Radiation

Radiation therapy—also called radiotherapy—is a highly targeted, highly effective way to destroy cancer cells in the breast that may be left following surgery. Radiation can reduce the risk of breast cancer recurrence by about 70 percent. It has an important place in your treatment analysis.

Despite what many people fear, radiation therapy is relatively easy to tolerate. Side effects are typically limited to the treated area and can be best described as a severe sunburn. There are special creams that will help mitigate this condition. In addition, fatigue often follows radiation. Unfortunately it can last for months. More information on overcoming fatigue is found in "#14 Overcome Fatigue and Nausea" in chapter 7, "The 50 Essential Things You Can Do."

A recent study questioned the value of radiation following mastectomy. I was sharing this news with Stephen, a radiation oncologist, who said he doubted the validity of the research. Then he added, "Look, Greg, neither of us has the training or the knowledge to interpret the quality of this evidence. I will keep radiating."

I know Stephen well. He is a loving doctor, devoted to doing God's will in this world. Even though he has a vested financial interest in radiation therapy, I sense he is driven to continue radiating patients more out of a genuine desire to help, even when he may not know with certainty what may or may not be the right thing to do. I am a believer in targeted radiation therapy.

Chemotherapy

Chemotherapy treatment employs specialized medicines to weaken, and hopefully to destroy, cancer cells. This includes cells at the original cancer site and other cancer cells that may have spread to another part of the body. Chemotherapy, often shortened to just chemo, is a systemic therapy, which means it affects the whole body by going through the bloodstream.

There are many chemotherapy medicines. In most cases, a combination of two or more medicines will be used as chemotherapy treatment for breast cancer.

Medical oncologists believe chemotherapy has a place in:

- Early-stage invasive breast cancer to get rid of any cancer cells that may be left behind after surgery in order to reduce the risk of recurrence

- Advanced-stage breast cancer to destroy or damage the cancer cells as much as possible

- In some cases, before surgery to shrink the cancer

More detailed treatment recommendations and analysis appear later in this book at "#7 Understand Your Conventional Treatment Options" in chapter 7, "The 50 Essential Things You Can Do." By themselves, conventional treatments are not a source of health and healing. Instead, they assist the body's natural healing capacity. One treatment in particular, surgery, has a role in most breast cancer journeys. See the next chapter of this book for further exploration of these options.

4

Caution Signs on the Incredible Journey

Surgery: Preparation and Timing

Presurgery Preparations

Consider the following strategies to prepare for surgery:

1. In the weeks leading up to surgery, eat well, incorporating plenty of fruits and vegetables into your diet.

2. Take time to decrease your stress levels, to exercise, and to relax.

3. Practice a daily visualization. Envision the tumor "presenting well" to the surgeon. Imagine the minimal loss of blood during surgery. See the incision healing quickly and completely.

If you choose to have breast reconstruction, make it a richer experience by exploring what else you can bring into your life at this time. How can this procedure be a turning point for you in a journey to a more fulfilling future? Clearly, breast surgery is a traumatic event. But your interpretation of it and how you choose to react to it will make all the difference.

When to Schedule Your Surgery

If you are premenopausal, schedule your breast surgery during the latter half of your menstrual cycle, when progesterone levels are highest.

There is excellent evidence to suggest that lower rates of recurrence correlate with surgery in the last two weeks of your normal cycle.

Radiation: Prepare for Side Effects

Side effects of external beam radiation therapy vary among patients. But by far the most common complaint is extreme tiredness. This fatigue often lasts weeks, even months, following radiation. Patients who experience fatigue after radiation sessions should honor the need for more rest while maintaining a moderate exercise program. I encourage you to do everything possible to be certain you remain reasonably active in spite of the fatigue.

Another common side effect of radiation therapy is called neutropenia. This is a drop in white blood cell counts. It is often accompanied by loss of appetite, also a common side effect in patients who have radiation therapy. By maintaining a healthful diet and adhering to a nutritional supplement program, you will minimize these effects.

Near the end of radiation treatment, many women experience swelling of the breast, a feeling of heaviness in the breast, or a sunburn-type appearance of the breast skin. These side effects usually disappear after six months. In addition, the breast skin may become moist. Wearing loose-fitting cotton clothing that breathes, avoiding constricting bras, and exposing the skin to air—but not direct sunlight—helps in healing more quickly. Bathing or showering in warm water rather than in hot water is recommended.

In most cases, the breast will look and feel the same after radiation therapy is completed, though it may be more firm. In rare cases, radiation therapy may cause changes in the breast size. Breasts may become larger due to fluid buildup or smaller due to tissue changes.

Radiation therapy of the axillary, or underarm, lymph nodes may result in lymphedema, which is a chronic swelling of the arm. Simple arm exercises such as the windmill rotation and other activities help prevent and manage lymphedema.

Finally, if you are pregnant, do not undergo radiation therapy, due to possible harm to the fetus.

Chemotherapy: Be Skeptical

Chemotherapy is the number one and most dangerous cause of over-treatment in breast cancer. It is dangerous, even when administered by the most experienced oncologist. I wish to make it clear that I am very cautious, even skeptical, about chemotherapy. I want you to know of my belief—some have called it a bias—in order to balance it with your own research and convictions regarding your treatment choices.

The guiding dictum of the Hippocratic oath is "First, do no harm." Chemotherapy does not measure up to this standard. Simply put, the goal of chemotherapy is to harm cancer cells by poisoning them in order to disrupt their ability to grow and multiply. Sometimes, in some cases of cancer, it works.

However, in this process, your host defense system is typically compromised and, at high doses, often irreparably damaged. Further, tumors that initially respond to treatment frequently develop a resistance to these toxic drugs. And while a tumor may respond a second time, the response is often at a much lower level of effectiveness.

Worse, with longer-term treatment, the body is typically weakened to a point where less-invasive alternatives have little chance to effectively rebuild immune function, extend life, or yield quality-of-life gains.

That said, let me also state that chemotherapy does have its place. Good science shows chemotherapy to be efficacious in producing long-term remission in most cases of Hodgkin's disease, acute lymphocytic leukemia, and testicular cancer. Chemotherapy is also shown to be effective in a handful of relatively rare, mainly childhood cancers including Burkitt's lymphoma, lymphosarcoma, and choriocarcinoma. Used with surgery and/or radiation therapy, chemotherapy plays a role in the successful treatment of Wilms' tumor, Ewing sarcoma, rhabdomyosarcoma, and retinoblastoma.

In addition, research shows chemotherapy to be effective in extending life by several months in many cases of ovarian cancer and small-cell lung cancer. However, chemotherapy by itself does not produce a cure. Further, quality of life typically suffers.

Sadly, adjuvant chemotherapy has become the standard of care for breast cancer. I call this sad because the evidence is simply not conclusive. At best, there may be a very small statistical advantage, at most a 2 to 4 percent gain, in survival rates for those who receive chemotherapy. But this small gain must be weighed against the very real potential for collateral damage caused by the same treatment. The single most common long-term problem is impairment of the heart function. In other words, while chemotherapy may seem to marginally increase survival rates, it substantially increases the risk of other potentially serious lifelong health problems.

For postmenopausal women with breast cancer, a statistically stronger case can be made for the hormone blocker raloxifene, now the preferred choice over tamoxifen. However, both these drugs have been linked to other health problems, including blood clots, stroke, and increases in endometrial cancer, uterine cancer, and liver cancer.

The hormone blockers are perhaps best suited to a narrow group of high-risk premenopausal breast cancer patients. The goal there is to reduce the risk of cancer spreading to the second breast. Evidence suggests the hormone blockers help. However, balance this against the evidence discussed in "#26 Take One Low-Dose Aspirin Each Day," in chapter 7, "The 50 Essential Things You Can Do."

Chemotherapy's one other area of limited success is colon cancer. There is still no conclusive evidence of its effectiveness except after lymph node involvement. Sadly, once again, even though the clinical evidence is at best mixed, the current Western practice says to treat virtually all cases of colon cancer with chemotherapy.

After studying this carefully for over a decade, I believe oncologists in the Western tradition are administering chemotherapy to more patients, across a wider spectrum of malignant disease, based on the hope it may show results. The cancer community has tended to extrapolate their narrow successes and consider nearly all patients, especially those with metastatic or recurrent cancer, as candidates for chemotherapy. All this to the exclusion of high-level nutrition, exercise, and mind-body regimens.

In short, those are my concerns about chemotherapy and its overuse. It is my belief that chemotherapy, under its current formulations, only rarely has a place in breast cancer care. I consider this an urgent warning to patients everywhere. I ask you to understand clearly, through your own independent research, what chemotherapy can be expected to do and what it cannot be expected to accomplish. Then make your own decision.

Science says, "Show me the data." The data says that, beyond the cancers mentioned above, there is no proof of chemotherapy's effectiveness in the form of large-scale randomized clinical trials. The unvarnished truth is the widespread use of chemotherapy is not based on convincing scientific data. Even in those cancers where some outcomes can be observed, current chemotherapy regimens alone fail to produce a cure, a longer life, or an improved quality of life. It is the multifaceted integrated cancer care approach emphasized throughout this book that is crucial to understand and implement.

Having stated my very real and urgent reservations, I need to state that chemotherapy may be right for you. One important aspect of any treatment's success is the belief both the doctor and the patient bring to the process. It's understandable that many oncologists believe in chemotherapy based on tumor response, or shrinkage. Theoretically, it makes sense. If you can reduce the tumor burden, perhaps the body can rebuild immune function.

From the patient's viewpoint, it is also understandable. Because chemotherapy is widely accepted and supported by the medical community, because insurance will reimburse for its administration, and because billions of cancer research dollars are invested in investigating this treatment modality, it comes with a great deal of upfront cultural support. With all that evidence, it seems believable.

If you do choose this therapy, I urge you to use extreme caution in approving high-dose chemotherapy. There are now dozens of studies on the use of high-dose chemotherapy across a broad spectrum of cancers. The results are universally disappointing. There are simply very few studies that show better outcomes with high-dose chemotherapy compared to those receiving lower-dose chemotherapy. This data directly challenges earlier studies and widely held assumptions regarding increased survival rates with higher doses.

But there is a middle ground you could choose. Fractionated-dose chemotherapy, smaller doses infused over an extended period of time, may be an option. The toxic effects of the drugs are typically minimized because the lower doses do not create massive systemic toxicity. In fact, there exists an increasing body of evidence from Europe that low-dose chemotherapy appears to stimulate immune function. Although most conventionally trained Western oncologists dismiss this evidence, I predict this homeopathic, less-is-more approach may become more widely accepted.

Finally, if you choose to undergo chemotherapy or have already had chemotherapy, study carefully "#21 Adopt This Nutritional Strategy" and "#25 Determine Your Nutritional Supplement Program," in chapter 7, "The 50 Essential Things You Can Do." Start strengthening and rebuilding your immune system immediately.

In summary, when you consider conventional medical treatments for breast cancer, I beg of you to consider the side effects, both short-term and long-term. And once treatment is started, if you are debilitated, confined to bed, and unable to eat, you not only have every right but also the responsibility to call a halt. Even in the face of threats and warnings from medical providers, continuing or stopping treatment is your personal choice.

In the final analysis, the vast majority of conventional breast cancer treatments do not cure by themselves. My general guidance is: Surgery, yes. Radiation, maybe. Chemotherapy, no—or at least be skeptical, very skeptical.

I ask you to be certain you carefully consider the balance between treating illness and creating health. Consider the whole.

Mammography: Time for a New Screening Protocol

Despite the loud protests of most breast cancer organizations and advocacy groups, the U.S. Preventive Services Task Force got it right. You don't need as many mammograms as you are getting!

Previous standards stated that women should be screened annually from the age of forty onward. A furor arose when the Task Force updated its recommendation on breast cancer screening in November 2009, advising that women between forty and forty-nine years old should not have annual mammograms.

Overtreatment in breast cancer is epidemic, a toxic tragedy that leaves the health of hundreds of thousands of women compromised for the remainder of their lives. The overtreatment starts with overdiagnosis in early screening for breast cancer.

It is my opinion that sometime in the early 1970s, leaders of the American medical profession and the largest cancer advocacy group came to the belief that the best way to keep people healthy was to instill fear. They helped create a culture in which people would be encouraged to go to their doctor to be screened for illnesses and conditions they did not even suspect they had. And today the list of tests is long, expensive, and invasive. Many of these tests routinely expose healthy people to treatment they do not need.

Breast cancer screening is unequalled in its unquestioned cultural acceptance. On the surface, the logic of screening for breast cancer seems unassailable. A mammogram can pick up lesions as small as half a centimeter, a size that you are usually not able to feel. The test is able to detect up to 85 percent of all breast cancers. This compares favorably with a Canadian best-practices study that showed that an experienced physician can detect up to 92 percent of breast cancers through a clinical breast exam. In short, screening for breast cancer seems to make sense.

But the screening is not without significant shortcomings and health risks. With mammography, there are some weak points:

- If a woman has dense breasts, a lump is typically not visible.
- In women under fifty years of age, at least 25 percent of the tumors will be missed.
- In women with smaller breasts, the screening is even less accurate.

According to Dr. Susan Love, mammograms will miss cancers between 9 and 20 percent of the time. And if nothing is found, women are given a false sense of security that all is well.

There's more. Approximately 5 percent of all mammograms read as positive for cancer. Of that number, 97.5 percent will be false positives. This means no cancer is present. In other words, out of every one thousand mammograms, fifty are read as positive, but only one or two will actually turn out to be breast cancer.

Another study found that women who had their mammograms during the last two weeks of their menstrual cycle were twice as likely to have false negative results. This means the cancer was missed.

The point is, mammograms are simply not conclusive. Yet we treat them as the gold standard of breast cancer screening.

Early screening brings a host of related risks, of which women worldwide still remain uninformed. Radiation from routine mammography poses significant cumulative risks of initiating and promoting breast cancer. Contrary to conventional assurances that radiation exposure from mammography is minimal and tolerable, we have known for at least forty years that the premenopausal breast is highly sensitive to radiation. Each exposure increases breast cancer risk, resulting in at least a cumulative 10 percent increased risk over ten years of premenopausal screening.

Mammography also poses a risk from breast compression. In his landmark book, *The Politics of Cancer*, Samuel S. Epstein, MD, reminds us that as early as 1928, physicians were warned to handle "cancerous breasts with care for fear of accidentally disseminating cells" and spreading cancer. Mammography requires tight and often painful compression of the breast, particularly in premenopausal women. Experts have warned that compression may lead to distant and lethal spread of malignant cells by rupturing small blood vessels in or around small, as-yet-undetected breast cancers.

Mammography is simply not reliable. Falsely negative readings are especially common in premenopausal women. This is due to the dense and highly glandular structure of their breasts and increased proliferation late in their menstrual cycle. Missed cancers are also common in postmenopausal women on estrogen replacement therapy, as about 20 percent develop breast densities that make their mammograms as difficult to read as those of premenopausal women.

Of greater concern is the proliferation of false positive readings. Mistakenly diagnosed cancers are particularly common in premenopausal women and also in postmenopausal women on estrogen replacement therapy. This results in needless anxiety, more mammograms, and unnecessary biopsies. For women with multiple high-risk factors, including a strong family history of breast cancer, prolonged use of hormone-based contraceptives, and early menarche, the very groups of women most strongly urged to have annual mammograms, the cumulative risk of false positives increases to "as high as 100 percent" over a decade's screening, according to Epstein.

The science says early detection of ductal carcinoma in situ does not reduce mortality.

The major risks of mammography add up to massive overdiagnosis and subsequent overtreatment. The widespread and virtually unchallenged acceptance of this early screening has resulted in a dramatic increase in the diagnosis of ductal carcinoma in situ (DCIS), a preinvasive cancer. DCIS is usually recognized as microcalcifications and generally treated by lumpectomy plus radiation or even mastectomy followed by chemotherapy.

However, some 80 percent of all DCIS cases never become invasive even if left untreated. Furthermore, the breast cancer mortality from DCIS is the same, approximately 1 percent, both for women diagnosed and treated early and for those diagnosed later following the development of invasive cancer.

That is startling and seems counterintuitive. But allow me to repeat for clarity. The science says early detection of ductal carcinoma in situ does not reduce mortality.

Mammograms are X-rays. They expose women to doses of radiation that are cumulative over time. The result is that a test meant to detect breast cancer actually increases one's risk of developing breast cancer. It can take up to forty years for cancer to show up following exposure to radiation. This clearly means that for women under fifty years old, annual mammograms increase the risk of developing breast cancer. This exposure to radiation is particularly important for women with a family history of breast cancer. These women are already at risk, high risk. Using diagnostic tools that increase the risk of developing breast cancer is an obvious case of overtreatment. Sadly, this is the norm in American medicine.

Less Is More

When we started our work at the Cancer Recovery Group more than a quarter century ago, I blindly followed medical orthodoxy. I believed the mantra, "The best protection is early detection." I was quick to say that all we did was in addition to, not in place of, conventional cancer care. I too eagerly urged all women to get mammograms beginning at age forty. I even endorsed younger women to use mammography if there was any suspicion of a lump in the breast. It was a mistake.

Much less invasive and nontoxic clinical breast examinations coupled with breast self-exams produce equal results.

Studies have subsequently shown that screening mammography does reduce the death rate in women over fifty years of age by approximately 30 percent. Early detection in this age group works. However, much less invasive and nontoxic clinical breast examinations coupled with breast self-exams produce equal results.

What is more worrisome are new studies that show that in women under fifty, screening mammography can increase the death rate from breast cancer by up to 50 percent. The main reason is because these women accumulate radiation toxicity. Even more, other studies show screening mammography leads to more frequent diagnosis and aggressive treatment of breast cancer. The studies also show this aggressive screening and treatment does not decrease overall breast cancer mortality.

These facts have now led me to recommend the following to the women who come to us for guidance on early screening for breast cancer:

For women under fifty years old:

- Employ annual clinical breast examinations and monthly breast self-examinations as your primary early detection protocol.

- Once a year, every year, without fail, schedule an appointment with your healthcare provider to perform a clinical breast examination. We recommend you schedule it on or near your birthday.

- Once a month, every month, without fail, set aside fifteen minutes to conduct a thorough breast self-examination. We recommend you schedule it on the first day of menstruation.

- Schedule a mammogram only if needed for diagnosis of a suspected lump. Even then, be sure to schedule that mammogram within the first fourteen days of your menstrual cycle.

- In addition, you may wish to employ annual thermography screening between the ages of thirty and fifty. This technology employs non-invasive digital infrared imaging to detect and analyze temperature variations in the breast, thought by many to be among the earliest signs of breast cancer.

- If you are between the ages of twenty and thirty, consider a thermogram every two years in addition to your monthly breast self-examinations.

For women over fifty years old:

- Employ annual clinical breast examinations and monthly breast self-examinations as your primary early detection protocol.

- Once a year, every year, without fail, schedule an appointment with your healthcare provider to perform a clinical breast examination. We recommend you schedule it on or near your birthday.

- Once a month, every month, without fail, set aside fifteen minutes to conduct a thorough breast self-examination. We recommend you schedule it on the first day of your period if you are still menstruating.

- Schedule a mammogram if you discover a lump. Even then, be sure to schedule that mammogram within the first fourteen days of your menstrual cycle if you are still menstruating.

- Employ mammography screening every other year.

- Consider thermography screening on alternate years.

- If a positive result comes back from the thermogram, schedule a mammogram.

I have come to understand mammography screening as an unreliable, mistake-riddled, profit-driven technology. In striking contrast, annual clinical breast examination by a trained health professional, together with monthly breast self-examination, is safe, at least as effective, and lower in cost.

Robert Aronowitz, MD, of the University of Pennsylvania points out in an op-ed in the *New York Times*, "You need to screen 1,900 women in their 40s for 10 years in order to prevent one death from breast cancer. And in the process you will have generated more than 1,000 false-positive screens and all the overtreatment they entail."

Claims for the benefit of screening mammography in reducing breast cancer mortality are based on eight international, controlled trials involving about five hundred thousand women. However, a meta-analysis of these trials revealed that only two, based on sixty-six thousand postmenopausal women, were adequately randomized to allow statistically valid conclusions. Based on these two trials, the authors concluded, "There is no reliable evidence that screening decreases breast cancer mortality—not even a tendency towards an effect." Accordingly, the authors determined that there is no longer any justification for wide-scale screening mammography.

Allow me to briefly lay out some statistics. Even assuming that high-quality screening of a population of women between the ages of fifty and sixty-nine would reduce breast cancer mortality by up to 25 percent, yielding a reduced relative risk of 0.75 percent, the chances of any individual woman benefiting are remote. For women in this age group, about 4 percent are likely to develop breast cancer annually. Approximately one in four of these women, or 1 percent overall, will die from this disease. Thus the three quarters of 1 percent relative risk applies to this 1 percent of women. This means that 99.75 percent of the women screened by mammography are unlikely to benefit. Astonishing, isn't it? But mammography is still considered the gold standard.

Annual clinical breast examination combined with monthly breast self-examination is a safe and effective alternative to mammography.

Annual clinical breast examination combined with monthly breast self-examination is a safe and effective alternative to mammography.

That most breast cancers are first recognized by women themselves was admitted in 1985 by the American Cancer Society, the leading advocate of routine mammography for all women over the age of forty: "We must keep in mind the fact that at least 90 percent of the women who develop breast carcinoma discover the tumors themselves." Furthermore, as previously shown, "training [women to do self-examinations] increases reported breast self-examination frequency, confidence, and the number of small tumors found."

A pooled analysis of several studies showed that women who regularly performed breast self-examinations detected their cancers much earlier and with fewer positive nodes and smaller tumors than women failing to examine themselves. Plus, breast self-examinations also enhance earlier detection of missed cancers, especially in premenopausal women.

Let's be clear. The effectiveness of breast self-exam critically depends on careful training by skilled professionals. Further, confidence in self-exams is enhanced with annual clinical breast examinations by an experienced professional using consistent techniques. And finally, this strategy requires discipline.

Every month, a breast self-exam; every year, a clinical breast exam. If a woman cannot or will not meet that standard of discipline, the entire process stands in jeopardy.

The question of more screening extends to what have come to be known as the breast cancer genes, BRCA1 (breast cancer gene one) and BRCA2 (breast cancer gene two). Women who inherit a mutation in either of these genes have a higher-than-average risk of developing breast cancer and ovarian cancer.

The function of the BRCA genes is to keep breast cells growing normally and to prevent any cancer cell growth. When these genes contain the mutations that are passed from generation to generation, they do not function normally, and breast cancer risk increases. Abnormal BRCA1 and BRCA2 genes may account for between 5 and 10 percent of all breast cancers.

Should you choose to undergo genetic testing to find out your status? A genetic test involves giving a blood sample that can be analyzed to pick up any abnormalities in these genes. Testing for these abnormalities is not done routinely, but it may be considered on the basis of your family history and personal situation. But remember that most people who develop breast cancer have no family history of the disease.

Then the question must be raised, what do I do with this information? In other words, if the test is negative, am I home free, never having to be concerned about breast cancer again? And if it is positive, what does that mean I should do?

Whether negative or positive, we suggest you employ the breast health program described in this book.

Vitamin D supplementation along with monthly breast self-exams and annual clinical breast exams remain the foundation of your prevention program.

If your test results are positive, there are further steps you can employ. The most important are lifestyle choices—improving diet, incorporating exercise into your daily routine, managing stress, and more. You may also wish to schedule clinical breast examinations every six months rather than annually. However, we do not recommend mammography unless there is a suspicious lump.

Nor do we recommend taking a drug such as tamoxifen, which conventional oncologists prescribe as a method to prevent the spread of breast cancer. This drug simply has too many adverse side effects even for someone with a BRCA mutation.

And we certainly do not recommend preventive or prophylactic surgical removal of your breasts before cancer has formed. Yet, sadly, there are physicians who routinely recommend this procedure.

In short, screening for the breast cancer gene is an individual choice. But no matter what the result, please maintain the breast health program we are offering in this book.

Mammography and genetic testing are vivid examples of the recommendations of powerful global medical technology and pharmaceutical industries instilling fear in unsuspecting women. In addition, the breast cancer advocacy establishment is complicit in keeping the fear alive. And the fervor is fanned by the mainstream media, which benefits from millions of dollars of advertising from all of these organizations.

In my opinion, genetic testing currently has very limited use in breast cancer screening. Plus, screening mammography should be phased out in favor of annual clinical breast examinations and monthly breast self-examinations. Employ diagnostic mammography when a suspicious clinical breast examination calls for further analysis. Such action is all the more critical and overdue in view of the evidence that screening mammography simply does not lead to decreased breast cancer mortality.

It is my conviction that this less-is-more breast cancer screening protocol must replace the massive overuse of mammography. This is the first necessary shift in the evolving breast cancer care model. Current annual mammography guidelines are exposing nearly all American women to exceedingly high levels of radiation. It's part of the toxic tragedy that is making us sicker—and poorer.

5

The Vitamin D Promise

Actual Prevention, Not Early Detection

AT CURRENT RATES, ONE IN TWO MEN and one in three women will be diagnosed with cancer in their lifetime. Breast cancer will account for the single most common diagnosis among women.

Here's the good news: we can now prevent nearly 80 percent of all breast cancers. Not early detection or early intervention, but prevention! That is a huge promise. It's real. It's vitamin D.

If you have followed the nutritional supplement field, you know I am required by law to say that these statements have not been evaluated by the U.S. Food and Drug Administration. Further, I am required to note that vitamin D supplements are not intended to diagnose, treat, cure, or prevent any disease. But what I can say is, do the research and decide for yourself. Here are the facts.

A Basic Understanding

It all starts naturally with our own body's ability to manufacture vitamin D.

The single most important thing every person should know about vitamin D is that the skin naturally produces a form of it, vitamin D_3 cholecalciferol (pronounced koh-luh-kal-SIF-uh-rawl)—a fact that has profound implications for the human condition. Technically not a vitamin, vitamin D is actually a hormone that interacts with more than two thousand genes, about 10 percent of the human genome.

Extensive research has implicated vitamin D deficiency as a major factor in the pathology of at least fourteen varieties of cancer, most notably breast and prostate cancer, as well as several other diseases.

Please understand that vitamin D is something we all need but nearly all of us lack in adequate amounts. And it's affecting our health.

Please understand that vitamin D is something we all need but nearly all of us lack in adequate amounts. And it's affecting our health.

The Science

Since 2005, cancer has become the leading cause of death for people under the age of eighty-five in America. Cancer now accounts for nearly one in every four deaths in the United States each year. It has also become the single leading cause of death worldwide. But scientific studies suggest that about three-fourths of those cancer deaths could be avoided! Statistics show that two thirds of the deaths that occurred in 2010 alone, for example, were related to lifestyle choices, such as tobacco use, obesity, physical inactivity, and poor nutrition and therefore could be prevented.

Enter vitamin D. Science shows that vitamin D hinders inappropriate cell division and metastasis, decreases blood vessel formation around tumors, and regulates proteins that influence tumor growth. It also enhances the immune system's ability to fight cancer and promotes the efficacy of several chemotherapeutic medicines.

In some of the most impressive research ever, studies conducted at the Creighton University School of Medicine in Nebraska have revealed that supplementing with vitamin D and calcium can reduce the risk of breast cancer by an astonishing 77 percent. This research provides strong new evidence that vitamin D is the single most effective preventive against breast cancer, far outpacing the benefits of any cancer drug known to modern science. Here's a portion of the Creighton press release:

Most Americans and others are not taking enough vitamin D, a fact that may put them at significant risk for developing cancer, according to a landmark study conducted by Creighton University School of Medicine.

The four-year, randomized study followed 1,179 healthy, post-menopausal women from rural eastern Nebraska. Participants taking calcium, as well as a quantity of vitamin D_3 nearly three times the U.S. government's Recommended Daily Amount (RDA) for middle-age adults, showed a dramatic 60 percent or greater reduction in cancer risk than women who did not get the vitamin.

The results of the study, conducted between 2000 and 2005, were reported in the June 8 [2007] online edition of the *American Journal of Clinical Nutrition*.

"The findings are very exciting. They confirm what a number of vitamin D proponents have suspected for some time but that, until now, have not been substantiated through clinical trial," said principal investigator Joan Lappe, Ph.D., R.N., Creighton professor of medicine and holder of the Criss/Beirne Endowed Chair in the School of Nursing. "Vitamin D is a critical tool in fighting cancer as well as many other diseases."

Research participants were all 55 years and older and free of known cancers for at least 10 years prior to entering the Creighton study. Subjects were randomly assigned to take daily dosages of 1,400–1,500 mg supplemental calcium; 1,400–1,500 mg supplemental calcium plus 1,100 IU of vitamin D; or placebos. National Institutes of Health funded the study.

Over the course of four years, women in the calcium/vitamin D3 group experienced a 60 percent decrease in their cancer risk than the group taking placebos.

On the premise that some women entered the study with undiagnosed cancers, researchers then eliminated the first-year results and looked at the last three years of the study. When they did that, the results became even more dramatic with the calcium/vitamin D_3 group showing a startling 77 percent cancer risk reduction.

In the three-year analysis, there was no statistically significant difference in cancer incidence between participants taking placebos and those taking just calcium supplements.

Through the course of the study, 50 participants developed nonskin cancers, including breast, colon, lung and other cancers.

Lappe said further studies are needed to determine whether the Creighton research results apply to other populations, including men, women of all ages, and different ethnic groups.

Please grasp the implications of this study. Over four years, the group receiving the calcium and vitamin D supplements showed a 60 percent decrease in cancer. When you discard the first year for margin of error, the study reveals an impressive 77 percent reduction in cancer attributable solely to vitamin D supplementation.

These astonishing effects were achieved on what many nutritionists consider to be a low dose of vitamin D. Exposure to sunlight, which creates even more vitamin D in the body, was not tested or considered. Plus the quality of the calcium supplements was likely not as high as it could have been. It was calcium carbonate and not high-grade calcium malate or aspartate.

when vitamin D levels are low, cancer deaths are relatively high; when vitamin D levels are high, cancer deaths are relatively low. Today, more than nine hundred scientific studies link vitamin D deficiency with breast cancer.

Beyond this groundbreaking study, additional research demonstrates vitamin D to be an effective cancer preventive. The science shows women who are vitamin D deficient have a 222 percent increased risk for developing breast cancer. Numerous studies have shown an inverse correlation between breast cancer mortality and vitamin D levels—when vitamin D levels are low, cancer deaths are relatively high; when vitamin D levels are high, cancer deaths are relatively low. Today, more than nine hundred scientific studies link vitamin D deficiency with breast cancer.

But the cancer community has been reluctant and slow to respond. Now I am asking you to study the evidence and decide for yourself. As you study, please consider the opinion of the experts, esteemed professionals in vitamin D research:

Cedric Garland, DPH, an adjunct professor for the Department of Family and Preventive Medicine at the University of California at San Diego, states, "Breast cancer is a disease so directly related to vitamin D deficiency that a woman's risk of contracting the disease can be 'virtually eradicated' by elevating her vitamin D status to what scientists consider to be natural blood levels."

Dr. Michael F. Holick, PhD, MD, author of *The Vitamin D Solution*, reports that there is an incredible potential opportunity to prevent breast cancer simply by increasing the supply of vitamin D in the body through supplements.

Anthony Norman, PhD, professor of biochemistry and biomedical sciences at the University of California at Riverside states that the majority of scientists believe that the currently recommended daily intake of vitamin D (between 200 IU and 600 IU) is not enough. "There is a wide consensus among scientists that the relative daily intake of vitamin D should be increased to 2,000 to 4,000 IU for most adults."

Tracey O'Connor, MD, an oncologist at Roswell Park Cancer Institute in Buffalo, New York, states she is now having all her patients supplement with vitamin D.

Since vitamin D carries no risk unless taken at enormously high amounts, it can only benefit both people who are already healthy as well as those who are sick. Those with debilitating diseases have been found to be the most deficient in vitamin D, indicating a clear correlation between deficiency and the onset of disease. For example, Dr. O'Connor points out that among women with breast cancer, about 80 percent are vitamin D deficient.

An Opportunity Missed

A wide range of vitamin D experts including those at the Cancer Recovery Group believed the opportunity for a breakthrough might be possible when the governments of Canada and the United States commissioned an Institute of Medicine (IOM) review on vitamin D recommendations. After three years of study, the institute's Food and Nutrition Board (FNB) issued a report on November 30, 2010, saying it had revised its recommendations made thirteen years previously on dietary reference intakes for vitamin D and calcium for Americans and Canadians.

The committee, consisting of more than a dozen panelists, recommended that most Americans and Canadians up to age seventy need no more than 600 IU of vitamin D per day to maintain health. It also stated that those seventy-one and older may need as much as 800 IUs.

The FNB claimed in its news release that it reviewed nearly one thousand published studies and testimonies from scientists. It said many studies yielded conflicting and mixed results on the effects of vitamin D on many important health conditions, including cancer, heart disease, autoimmune diseases, and diabetes, among others. The report concluded that no solid evidence suggests that higher than the recommended dietary reference intakes are needed.

The report was a huge disappointment to the hundreds of us dedicated to the task of actually preventing cancer. The Cancer Recovery Group responded to the new recommendations, saying in a news release that "according to scientific studies, right now 70 percent of whites and 97 percent of African Americans are vitamin D deficient. And the evidence is overwhelming that vitamin D deficiency is directly linked to fourteen different cancers, most prominently breast and prostate cancer."

The FNB's report ignored research showing that in order to maintain adequate vitamin D levels, much higher doses of vitamin D must be consumed. Excellent research exists to support this position. Unfortunately, the recommendation was made by panelists, only a few of which had experience in vitamin D research. Even worse, the panel suppressed the findings of some of the world's most prominent vitamin D scientists, including our esteemed friends Cedric Garland, Michael Holick, and Anthony Norman.

Dr. John Cannell, MD, a vitamin D expert and director of the Vitamin D Council, pointed out that the IOM's recommendation that a baby and a pregnant woman need the same amount of vitamin D did not make any sense. He said his organization pressed the IOM to release the comments on vitamin D and health from fourteen vitamin D experts, which have not been released.

Cancer Recovery Group joined him with an online petition asking Harvey Fineberg, MD, PhD, president of the Institute of Medicine, to include the testimony of these esteemed scientists. Thereafter, we filed a Freedom of Information request with the Institute of Medicine. Sadly, there has been no response.

In a follow-up statement, the FNB suggested that without "solid" evidence, it is risky to recommend high intake of vitamin D. It cited vitamin E as an example to suggest that high intake of vitamin D could lead to toxicity issues. (In the short term, vitamin E can help mitigate oxidative stress, but prolonged intake above 3,000 IU per day can interfere with the blood's ability to clot.)

The FNB statement may sound convincing to some people. But at the sunniest time of a summer day, exposure of the face and arms to the sun for fifteen to twenty minutes generates more than 10,000 IU of vitamin D in the body. And there is no toxicity issue in such a natural dose.

Your geographic latitude and your ancestry influence your body's ability to convert sunlight into vitamin D. People with dark skin have more difficulty making the vitamin. Persons living at latitudes north of the thirty-fifth parallel cannot obtain adequate levels of vitamin D naturally during the winter months because of the sun's angle.

The laboratory research is convincing to all but the most skeptical scientists. Here is just some of the overwhelming evidence:

- In animal studies, vitamin D_3 has repeatedly and definitively been shown to inhibit the growth of a variety of tumors including breast cancer.

- Even synthetic vitamin D–like molecules have prevented the equivalent of breast cancer in laboratory animals.

- Again in the lab, vitamin D$_3$ has been shown to inhibit the growth of new blood vessels that allow cancer cells to grow and spread. This process, called antiangiogenesis, has been heralded as a breakthrough.

There's more. For decades we have known of the evidence that women over fifty years of age who skimp on foods rich in vitamin D are more likely to develop breast cancer. The late Frank Garland, PhD, brother of Cedric, who also conducted vitamin D research at the University of California at San Diego, especially noted the anti-cancer protection of fish, because fatty fish is loaded with vitamin D.

In England, researchers from St. George's University of London found that local production of vitamin D directly in the breast reduces the risk for breast cancer. In fact, in women with low breast-tissue levels of vitamin D, the risk for breast cancer rose by an incredible 354 percent. The study went so far as to suggest that women may wish to sunbathe with their breasts exposed to enhance vitamin D production.

Dr. Edward Giovannucci, professor of nutrition and epidemiology at Harvard School of Public Health in Boston, Massachusetts, in a letter to the Cancer Recovery Group, wrote this in support of our vitamin D intake recommendations:

> Because most people do not get adequate vitamin D in typical diets, and because of the potential downsides of excessive sun exposure, most people may benefit from vitamin D supplements. Several groups are at risk for vitamin D deficiency or less-than-adequate intakes—in particular, the elderly, dark-skinned individuals, obese individuals, and those who avoid the sun. For those at a higher risk of vitamin D deficiency, a larger daily supplement dose, on the order of 3,000–4,000 IU, may be required to achieve adequate blood levels, which in my opinion are in the range of 30–40 ng/mL based on current knowledge.

John H. White, PhD, a physiology and medicine professor at McGill University in Montreal, concurred: "There is now substantial and compelling evidence that, in addition to its requirement for skeletal integrity, vitamin D sufficiency reduces the risk of development of a number of cancers, contributes to cardiovascular health, and stimulates immune response."

We also heard from Susan J. Whiting, PhD, a professor of nutrition and dietetics at the University of Saskatchewan in Saskatoon, Canada:

> We know from intake studies that people cannot get much more than 200 IU per day. There's not enough choice in the marketplace nor [adequate] levels in existing foods. That means almost everyone needs a supplement. One must realize that risk/benefit is not confined to high doses. Not taking enough is a risk.

William B. Grant, PhD, of the Sunlight, Nutrition, and Health Research Center (SUNARC) in San Francisco, California, offered these comments on the IOM's report:

> How could the IOM committee have set such low guidelines for vitamin D in light of the large body of evidence that vitamin D has important health benefits affecting risk of many types of disease? While the committee claimed it made a thorough review and assessment of over 1000 studies and reports . . . they ignored 49,000 other papers on vitamin D listed at *www.pubmed.gov*.
>
> Institute of Medicine, let the science speak. The laboratory evidence for vitamin D is at least as strong as that routinely accepted as "proof of concept" for dozens of cancer drugs. And the evidence from clinical trials is much stronger. The message is crystal clear: vitamin D regulates the expression of both genes and proteins connected with breast cancer.

The evidence of vitamin D's influence on key biological functions vital to health and well-being mandates that vitamin D no longer be ignored by our government, by the healthcare industry, or by individuals striving to achieve and maintain a greater state of health.

The evidence of vitamin D's influence on key biological functions vital to health and well-being mandates that vitamin D no longer be ignored by our government, by the healthcare industry, or by individuals striving to achieve and maintain a greater state of health.

Can vitamin D play a role in treating breast cancer, in addition to preventing it? Yes. The cancer-stopping potential of vitamin D in breast cancer patients has been well documented. Up to the point of massive differentiation, vitamin D receptors are present in breast cancer cells. This means these same cells are responsive to the anti-cancer effects of this vitamin. And that fact provides a potential game-changing breakthrough in breast cancer treatment.

Vitamin D supplements and vitamin D–rich foods including salmon, tuna, and fish oils all contribute to transitioning the breast cancer cells from a short-term threat into a long-term manageable condition. If a cell has already undergone malignant transformation, activated vitamin D can team up with other proteins to stimulate programmed death of abnormal cells, the process known as cell apoptosis.

There's more good news. A growing body of evidence shows that a higher intake of vitamin D may be helpful in the prevention and treatment of high blood pressure, fibromyalgia, diabetes, multiple sclerosis, rheumatoid arthritis, and other diseases.

Critics of vitamin D point to the potential for overdosing, resulting in toxic levels of the vitamin in the bloodstream. Symptoms of vitamin D toxicity include anorexia, disorientation, dehydration, fatigue, weight loss, weakness, and vomiting. One study demonstrated these effects when a single dose of 500,000 IU of vitamin D_3 was injected into a patient. A half million IU at once seems irrationally high and no doubt can result in toxicity. But numerous studies show levels of 10,000 IU per day to be safe. The fact is vitamin D toxicity is very rare.

As I previously noted, the skin produces approximately 10,000 IU of vitamin D in response to fifteen to twenty minutes of summer sun exposure. However, most people do not receive fifteen to twenty minutes of sun exposure daily. This is especially true in northern and southern latitudes during their winter months. When healthy adults and adolescents are regularly deprived of adequate sunlight exposure, research indicates that it's advisable to supplement with at least 2,000 units of vitamin D daily.

What does all this mean? It means you have a decision to make. It means that if you maintain adequate calcium levels and receive adequate natural sunlight exposure, you can reduce your chances of getting breast cancer by up to 77 percent. Or if you daily consume a high-quality calcium supplement and take premium vitamin D supplements such as those made from fish oil, you could easily have a greater than the 77 percent reduction recorded in the Creighton University study.

We now have hundreds of studies to show that most North Americans who live above the thirty-fifth parallel, a line that runs roughly from Los Angeles through Atlanta, Georgia, are deficient in vitamin D. That deficiency has been correlated with a host of diseases, most notably breast and prostate cancers.

In the early days of my work more than twenty-five years ago, the science was not there to support our common-sense claims regarding nutrition and exercise in integrated cancer care. Today, the scientific evidence is overwhelming, especially the evidence for vitamin D supplementation. But it is now ignored by our government. This is exceedingly frustrating and totally unacceptable.

Decide for yourself. I stand by the Cancer Recovery Group's recommendations for healthy adults to supplement with vitamin D at the rate of 2,000 IU per day, and 5,000 IU daily if you are dealing with a cancer diagnosis. See "#25 Determine Your Nutritional Supplement Program" in chapter 7, "The 50 Essential Things You Can Do" for further details.

This much I believe to be true: with vitamin D supplementation, we can now prevent nearly 80 percent of all breast cancers. This is actual prevention, not early detection or early intervention. And with vitamin D supplementation, we can assist in boosting the effectiveness of the treatment of breast cancer.

Those are huge promises. Vitamin D delivers.

Part Two

Integrated Breast Cancer Care

6

The Holistic Model

FROM THE MOMENT MY WIFE and I started what would become the Cancer Recovery Group, our approach has always been holistic. This means we recognize the central importance of integrating body, mind, and spirit—the physical, emotional, and spiritual components of health and well-being.

I have now come to understand the profound truth that health is much more than not being physically ill. We have also come to understand that breast cancer is much, much more than cells gone awry. This leads to an equally profound point of understanding: Surviving breast cancer is not simply about treating illness. It is primarily about creating wellness.

I have come to this deeply held belief based on extensive surveys and interviews with more than sixteen thousand cancer survivors. Along with a wonderful team of associates at the Cancer Recovery Group, we studied what went right with cancer patients—what led to survival.

Today, I can emphatically state: orthodox medical treatment alone does not maximize one's opportunity for breast cancer survival.

Having said that, I need to make clear that all I am suggesting is to be considered in addition to, not in place of, conventional medical care. That's what the term *integrated cancer care* means.

Evidence abounds that when a patient integrates complementary and even alternative approaches into a conventional biomedical cancer treatment program, it is very likely to result in better outcomes, reduced side effects, a greater sense of control, and much improved quality of life.

While the Cancer Recovery Group and our affiliate, Breast Cancer Charities of America, certainly support each individual's choices and decisions in treatment—be they strictly conventional, complementary, or alternative—we have become much more assertive in urging the integrated approach. Our work takes three forms:

- Educate. Help patients understand their diagnosis of breast cancer, the spectrum of treatment options, and what they can do to help themselves.

- Empower. Guide patients to actually implement these strategies in their breast cancer recovery journey, creating a new way of life.

- Encourage. Support by offering inspiration and hope that no matter how difficult, patients can survive and even thrive through the breast cancer experience.

Those are big promises. The integrated breast cancer care strategy makes good on those promises.

Up to this point, this book has given you primarily background information. Now I want us to examine and explore the implementation of this holistic strategy, to help you apply these ideas in simple, understandable steps. These ideas offer you a plan to get well and stay well for the remainder of your life, however long or short that time may be.

The end result is a unique body-mind-spirit approach to health and healing. These strategies improve the ability to deal rationally with a breast cancer diagnosis, make intelligent and informed choices in treatment, and mobilize all the resources available to you in the healing process.

In the end, the integrated cancer care strategy helps turn the crisis of breast cancer into a unique opportunity to live far more happily and healthfully than ever before.

Your Current State of Health

In the early years of our work, the Cancer Recovery Group looked to the cellular biology of cancer as the starting point. That was a mistake. Integrated cancer care is built on a platform that extends well beyond the tumor model.

Today, our starting point is to view each person's state of health as a result of the many interactive components of body, mind, and spirit. As I have stated, cell biology may be a component, but health is more often the result of a host of lifestyle choices. These include nutrition, exercise, attitudes, social support, and spirituality. This definition of health also includes the environment, the air we breathe, the water we drink, and especially environmental toxins and the sea of chemicals in which we live. Lifestyle also includes our psychological and emotional makeup and the way in which we process all the above factors.

Yes, cancer does involve genes and genetic mutations. But you and I possess the ability to switch on and off the expression of those genes. And we can accomplish this naturally.

In the current medical culture, there is a pervasive belief that genetics explains cancer and is the basis of a cancer cure. I hold in my hands a *New York Times* article that begins, "The hope to cure cancer rests with finding the rogue genes." Epigenetics, the study of processes that change cells but do not alter the actual DNA gene sequence, is touted as the next cancer breakthrough. Millions of research dollars are being spent to discover treatments that may turn off certain genetic cancer switches.

Yes, cancer does involve genes and genetic mutations. But you and I possess the ability to switch on and off the expression of those genes. And we can accomplish this naturally.

Even the preeminent leaders in the epigenetics field conclude and agree that lifestyle has a massive influence on disease prevention and treatment. In fact, lifestyle choices can reverse or control a variety of genetic predispositions. Some basic examples: If you smoke cigarettes, the chances are greater that your cells will be damaged and your lungs much more susceptible to cancer. Eat with nutritional intelligence, and chances are your cellular mutations will successfully self-resolve. Daily exercise absolutely changes your biochemistry, and this influences cellular biology. So do our emotional responses. The point is, lifestyle choices readily trigger epigenetic mechanisms that can assist you in resolving breast cancer and preventing its recurrence.

Let's be clear. Our starting point is not genes gone haywire; it is your state of health. So how is it? How healthy are you? If you step back and observe, you will see many complex influences working around and through you. And it's more than just physical well-being.

One way to assess your state of holistic well-being is to ask yourself a series of questions, holding yourself accountable for honest answers.

Physical Well-Being:

Do I truly practice high nutritional intelligence?

Do I exercise each day?

Do I seek health guidance from competent health guides?

Attitudinal Well-Being:

Do I believe my life is filled with possibilities or obstacles?

Do I see my happiness as a choice or as a condition dependent on circumstances?

Do I understand my beliefs and perceptions are the source of both my peace and my pain?

Emotional Well-Being:

Do I possess an awareness of my dominant emotional style?

Do I feel free to express my feelings, or do I keep a stiff upper lip?

Do I understand how to choose and manage my emotions?

Social Well-Being:

Do I feel a close connection with others?

Do I both give and receive attention?

Do I have someone with whom I can share everything?

Spiritual Well-Being:

Do I have a sense there is more, a divine part to life?

Do I have an intimate connection with the divine?

Do I know what to do to establish and strengthen that connection?

While certainly not exhaustive, this picture of one's state of health is central to an understanding of getting well again. The result of such an understanding is the ability to mobilize the whole person—body, mind, and spirit—not only to recover from breast cancer but also to achieve your best life now.

This holistic understanding is at odds with breast cancer orthodoxy. It takes us well beyond cell biology and is in stark contrast to the conventional medical approach that is the norm in Western medicine today. The biomedical understanding of health focuses exclusively on the physical dimensions of well-being and envisions our body as a machine. Disease is considered a malfunction of the machine.

Mobilize the whole person—body, mind, and spirit—not only to recover from breast cancer but also to achieve your best life now.

According to this disease model, breast cancer is a specific failure that can be remedied by correcting that failure. This worldview very logically leads to mechanical fixes that predominantly rely on surgery, radiation therapy, and chemotherapy.

Medical treatments certainly have a time and a place in many breast cancer recovery programs. However, I have come to understand that they are not to occupy the dominant place. Instead, after more than twenty-five years of study and experience, I now believe these treatments are temporary steps to allow the body the opportunity to alleviate the burden of breast cancer. Once the burden is lessened, the whole person can then go forward in the creation of health and healing.

This is viewed as a radical position, I know. I also believe it is totally accurate and completely trustworthy, the rational alternative to the sole use of increasingly toxic, invasive, and experimental cancer treatments.

A Different Kind of Illness

We have already briefly explored that breast cancer is a complex and multidimensional process. It has a wide spectrum of causes and influences including genetics, nutrition, stress, environment, and even emotions. Some of these causes are direct, some indirect.

The physical symptoms resulting from these causes are the cellular component of cancer. We can accurately think of cancer, at the cell level, as the mutation of genes resulting in the irregular growth of abnormal cells. The operative words here are *irregular* and *abnormal*.

Healthy cells of the body grow in predictable patterns. As they wear out, they are replaced in an orderly manner by just the right number of new healthy cells.

Cancerous cells grow in uncontrolled and unpredictable patterns. Their growth serves no useful biological purpose. They often threaten the entire body. The cells themselves are mutant, changed in ways that limit their function.

You have this cellular condition in your breast. It is one of more than one hundred types of cancers, each having its own site and distinguishing characteristics.

Another dimension of breast cancer is an inefficient immune system. Your understanding of this point is of vital importance, critical in the decision to do all you can to help yourself get well. Your immune system is the first and most powerful defense your body has against cancer. For years, you have periodically produced mutant cells that were potentially cancerous. In most cases, the immune system was there to clean up the problems. Now your immune system has ceased doing so in an efficient enough manner to ensure your health.

Rebuilding immune function is central to getting well and staying well. My loving intention is to give you specific steps to help you respond with maximum intelligence to this diagnosis and to help you rebuild your self-healing functions. The basic action points are as follows:

1. Examine. Step back from the day-to-day pressures of your life to evaluate your current situation in its entirety.

2. Discover. Assess both current life issues that must be changed as well as future needs that must be met.

3. Plan. Create a simple plan to restore health and total well-being.

4. Implement. Work in partnership with health advisers who have your confidence. Begin a self-care plan to create whole-person well-being.

5. Review. Conduct quarterly reviews of your progress, making adjustments as necessary.

Taken together, these action points will play the central role in mobilizing all your healing options and capacities, both external and internal. You will then live vibrantly well for as long as you live. Living vibrantly well . . . that is a wonderful definition of health and healing.

When you make the decision to live vibrantly well, no matter what the state of your physical health, you have put the body-mind-spirit connection to work. It is real. It is powerful. When you use it in conjunction with prudent medical care, you can be assured you have created the optimum environment for healing. Your medical team will do all it can to fix the malfunctioning machine. Your task is to do all you can to create wellness and enhance your self-healing capacity.

Enhancing self-healing is accomplished through your own choices—your physical, emotional, and spiritual lifestyle. There is abundant authoritative, scientifically validated evidence that the immune system is profoundly influenced by lifestyle choices. Few people would argue that tobacco use, improper diet, and lack of exercise are obvious deterrents to maximum health. So is mismanaged toxic stress, which fills the body with adrenaline and cortisone derivatives, both known to inhibit immune function.

Something as basic as your emotional response to the communication of a cancer diagnosis is a factor. Most women receive the message "It's breast cancer" with pervasive fear. That fear can paralyze the recipient emotionally and psychologically at a time when intelligent action is required. And a spiritually toxic outlook after a breast cancer diagnosis can make a difficult situation a living hell. All these responses have a negative physiological impact on immune function.

The comprehensive integrated holistic emphasis of this book and the implementation of the strategies that flow from this approach should not be interpreted to be critical of the validity of truly scientific medicine. I do not encourage you to go back to the use of folk medicine, though I do have the utmost respect for the loving family doctor, the one who listens, shows compassion, and treats the whole person.

Many times over the last quarter century of our work, I have been asked to provide proof of my methods. The fact is, I do not have proof in the form of double-blind clinical research studies. But I can refer to a preponderance of evidence that points to the connection between nutrition, exercise, and social support and recovery from cancer. We have completed careful content analysis of sixteen-thousand-plus survivor surveys and interviews. I am keenly aware that some people do not equate this evidence with proof. But understand this: lack of double-blind studies is not equal to disproof.

Many widely accepted orthodox breast cancer treatment protocols are based on lack of complete proof.

Many widely accepted orthodox breast cancer treatment protocols are based on lack of complete proof. In fact, there is a long and sordid history of conventional treatments that prove to be not only disappointing but also dangerous. The drug Avastin is a prime example. Just a couple of years ago, the Food and Drug Administration gave this drug accelerated approval for breast cancer treatment. The approval was based on a single clinical trial. The result showed that Avastin, when added to standard chemotherapy, slowed the progression of tumors. However, it did not extend lives. So they had evidence but not proof.

Two follow-up trials by Genentech, the maker of Avastin, also found tumor progression was held at bay but for shorter periods of time. And once again, lives were not extended. Worse, some patients suffered serious and disabling side effects, including severe bleeding, stroke, heart problems, severe high blood pressure, and the perforation of the gastrointestinal tract. Approximately 1 percent of the clinical trial patients died from causes directly related to the drug.

Thankfully, the FDA advisory committee voted twelve to one that the drug's approval for breast cancer should be withdrawn. In Britain, the drug did not receive approval because of its lack of demonstrated benefit and survival time extension. However, the European Union ruled that the benefits outweighed the risks and gave it the go-ahead. Back in the United States, Genentech is in the process of demanding a hearing to argue the case for retaining Avastin's use in breast cancer treatment.

Proof? Not with Avastin. Evidence, scant evidence? Yes. But the FDA still gave approval, even though it was forced to rescind it. Better quality evidence exists for the anticancer properties of broccoli, raspberries, green tea, and a host of other natural foods. But because they cannot be patented, no clinical trials have been completed. There is no money in it. That is why it is so critically important for both public and private institutions to finance human studies on the link between foods, cancer prevention, and cancer treatment.

Even if there is only evidence, I ask you to join me in not waiting for those clinical trials. The breast cancer recovery diet we recommend here does not expose those who follow it to any risks. Instead, it produces health benefits that have a profound effect on cancer.

René Dubos, who discovered the first antibiotic put to medical use and is considered one of the great 20th-century leaders in medicine and ecology, may have said it best when, at the end of his career, he stated:

> I have always thought that the only trouble with scientific medicine is that it is not scientific enough. Modern medicine will become truly scientific only when patients and their medical teams learn to manage the forces of the body and the mind that operate via *vis medicatrix natureae [the healing power of nature]*.

That is exactly what I am attempting to help you do—manage the forces of the body, mind, and spirit that, when added to the forces of rational medical care, result in optimal health and healing.

If you have cancer today, you can't wait for years of clinical research to yield absolute proof of these points. So don't wait. You have nothing to lose and everything to gain.

Becoming proactive in creating your own health and healing will influence not only your quality of life but also your quantity of life. Integrate these principles with the best minimally invasive, least toxic treatments medicine has to offer. Therein you will find optimum success.

Believe this: breast cancer is indeed a different kind of illness that demands a different kind of response. Recovery demands your participation. For breast cancer patients determined to conquer this illness, that is very good news indeed.

No Such Thing as Hopeless

You may have been told, "Get your affairs in order," or "You have just a short time left," or a favorite of the medical community, "Your breast cancer is terminal." Don't believe it. Refuse to give in to that despair. Only God knows how long a person has to live.

In 1984, I was given thirty days to live. It was lung cancer. I'd previously had one lung removed. Four months after the surgery, the cancer was back. This time it was in my ribs and lymph system. The surgeon put his hand on my shoulder and said, "Greg, the tiger is out of the cage. Your cancer has come roaring back. I would give you about thirty days to live."

Part of the reason that surgeon was mistaken is that no health-care provider can predict a person's response to illness. After several days of believing I would die, I made a profound decision. I decided to live.

Please clearly understand what I am saying. By deciding to live, I made a decision to do all I could to triumph over the cancer. I determined to live each day I was given to the very best of my ability.

I chose not to focus on the blatant despair in the surgeon's words. I would instead adopt a stance of hopefulness. These decisions dramatically changed my experience of illness. They resulted not only in better days but many more days as well. I believe such a decision by you may result in a similar outcome in your breast cancer journey.

I deeply empathize with you and your health crisis. I have been there. I have been torn by some of the same emotions that now tear at you. I can identify with your fear and uncertainty. It is the most frightening time of your life.

Two paths are before you. One is marked by the road signs of passiveness and despair, the other by the guideposts of engagement and hope. You have a choice.

If you have been told that your time is limited, I encourage you to believe that life can still be a fulfilling adventure.

Choose to live life to the very fullest. Focus on the possibilities of life, not the problems of breast cancer. Affirm that each day is a good and perfect gift in spite of the circumstances of illness. Keep your thoughts on health, not on illness. In that intentional choice are the seeds of your health and healing. Water those seeds, not the weeds of dis-ease.

Without question, you can improve your potential for survival. What you do makes a significant difference. Believe it: there is no such thing as a hopeless situation.

The Road Map to Recovery

Between 1986 and 2008, Cancer Recovery Group interviewed and received surveys from more than sixteen thousand survivors of cancer. This group included all types of cancers, not just breast cancer.

These inspiring individuals, who possess no more courage or ability than you or I, teach some very powerful lessons from which breast cancer patients would be well served to learn. These ideas and practices have worked successfully for tens of thousands of other cancer patients, revealing the lessons and strategies that can be pivotal in your life and your health.

After the first five hundred interviews, it became clear that there were similar patterns to most of the individual experiences. For example, the vast majority of survivors do not believe they recovered their health by chance or by being passive. The triumphant patients worked for their wellness, earning it on a daily basis. Neither do most cancer survivors credit their doctors alone, or even primarily, for their recovery. Instead, these exceptional patients focused on personally mobilizing body, mind, and spirit in their quest for high-level wellness.

Consistent patterns emerged from the survivor interviews. In 1988, we first summarized and combined the lessons into an eight-strategy program. In 2006, after thousands of additional interviews, we further refined them into six easily understood concepts that anyone could implement. Today, through the various affiliates of Cancer Recovery Group, including Breast Cancer Charities of America, more than five million people have used these principles as a road map, a strategic plan to enhance their health and enrich their lives. I want the same for you.

The 6 Key Strategies

Before we come to the 50 Essential Things You Can Do, let's take an overview of the six basic approaches that cancer survivors have in common. Here is what emerged from the survivor interviews.

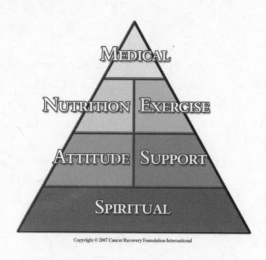

Copyright © 2007 Cancer Recovery Foundation International

You will immediately see how these strategies parallel our previous discussion in chapter 2, "The Sources of Health and Healing."

#1 Medical

More than 96 percent of cancer survivors start and complete at least one treatment program that is grounded in conventional medical care. Surgery, radiation therapy, chemotherapy, hormonal therapy, and immunotherapy—often in combination—are the orthodox treatments of choice.

The Cancer Recovery team was both surprised and encouraged by this. Orthodox treatments have a central role in cancer survival. The overwhelming majority of cancer survivors do embrace conventional Western medical treatment. This is an important message that must be heeded.

But there is a significant problem, an exceptionally troubling issue, that has become clear since we first started our work. It's the inconsistency in the medical treatment prescribed for similar diagnoses. I have already mentioned differences in breast cancer treatment in different parts of the country as an example. Although several well-designed studies have clearly demonstrated that breast conserving treatment (BCT) or lumpectomy for Stage I and II disease has the same success rate as mastectomy, the removal of the breast remains the predominant treatment.

There are also marked differences based on factors like the size of the city where patients live. The evidence in the Dartmouth Atlas work is clear: women in larger cities are more likely to receive BCT than those in rural areas, again despite the fact that the outcomes are statistically the same.

"I did my homework," shared Marti, a breast cancer patient from rural Colorado. "And I challenged the surgeon's recommendation [for mastectomy]. We even had an argument about the need for a sentinel node biopsy. I insisted on lumpectomy. And I had the science on my side."

Today, many more breast cancer patients are taking matters into their own hands, demanding full knowledge and explanation of treatment options. Thankfully, the amount of treatment information now available is significant. The key is questioning and demanding hard evidence regarding the effectiveness of suggested treatments, chemotherapy in early-stage breast cancer being the prime example. So while ninety-six out of one hundred patients still opt for conventional treatments, the treatment decision is more informed today than ever before.

Importantly, cancer survivors do not stop with conventional medical treatment. As you study the 50 Essential Things You Can Do (see chapter 7), you will see how breast cancer survivors take charge of the management of their entire medical program. They choose doctors in whom they have confidence, often researching their academic background and clinical record. Survivors tend to give consent only to treatment programs in which they have confidence and even a conviction. Plus, survivors aggressively integrate complementary and even alternative approaches with conventional medical care.

Breast cancer survivors are active patients, involved with each decision, making certain they are fully informed and understand each component of their treatment and recovery program. Conventional medicine, yes. Patient in control, even more.

#2 Nutrition

Following medical care, dietary changes are the most common strategy adopted by cancer survivors. The increasing importance of nutrition in cancer recovery has been one of the most significant shifts in the last decade.

Marissa was told by her doctor to eat whatever she wanted. "I knew intuitively that was not correct. In fact, fifty-one years of a high-fat diet prior to diagnosis was probably part of the reason I now had breast cancer. So I changed."

It's all so basic. View food as medicine. This means fundamental nutritional shifts:

- Eat whole foods.

- Minimize fat, salt, and sugar.

- Emphasize vegetables, fresh fruits, and whole grains

Among the survivors, the single major dietary shift is consuming foods that are less processed. Prepared foods, no matter how convenient, tend to deliver calories with less nutrition than their fresh counterparts. In practice, cancer survivors spend most of their grocery shopping time in the produce section of their local market.

Nutritional supplements, while clearly not taking the place of a whole-food diet, are widely employed by cancer survivors. While there exists a lack of consensus in actual practice, survivors recognize the role of vitamin, mineral, and herbal supplements in the management of breast cancer. Thankfully, science is currently producing evidence to support nutrition as a central element in cancer recovery. We will detail our recommendations in #21 of the 50 Essential Things You Can Do.

Cancer survivors eat with greater awareness. You can observe the marked increase in nutritional IQ in just the past ten years. Nutrition, not simply calories, has become the emerging battle cry of cancer patients in Western cultures. And survivors typically carry the attitude that diet is something they get to do, as opposed to have to do. High-level nutrition contributes significantly to breast cancer survival. Specific nutrition recommendations will be forthcoming later in this book.

#3 Exercise

Survivors engage in physical exercise virtually every day. Cancer Recovery Group was the very first cancer charity to document the benefits of exercise more than twenty years ago. Today, the science is catching up with the survivors' practices and confirming its efficacy.

Nearly nine out of ten cancer survivors surveyed affirm the role of regular physical exercise in their own journey. There are bikers, swimmers, joggers, and walkers—lots of walkers. A brisk thirty- to forty-minute walk each day, or strength training every other day, is ideal for many.

Carleen is now a thirteen-year breast cancer survivor. She shared, "My turning point? When I started to exercise, I started to get well again." It is an experience shared with hundreds of thousands of breast cancer survivors.

In our interviews, the most inspiring patients are those who started exercise programs even while confined to hospital beds or wheelchairs. In spite of physical limits, these people exercised. Believe it: physical exercise needs to be part of your breast cancer recovery program.

#4 Attitude

More than any other single practice, survivors embrace beliefs that generate attitudes that, in turn, create emotions that nurture healing. Allow me to repeat: beliefs precede attitudes, which result in emotions. This is the powerful mind-body connection.

Do beliefs and attitudes actually heal? Survivors see a direct link. They choose beliefs and attitudes about illness and wellness that empower. The most fundamental and empowering belief is that cancer does not mean death.

It's sad but true that much of the world still considers cancer and death to be synonymous. Survivors emphatically reject that belief; in fact, they stake their lives on it.

This does not translate into denial, some be-positive-against-all-evidence thinking. Nor is it just willpower. It's a warrior's attitude that survivors demonstrate. There is a marked tough-mindedness in the cancer survivor community, a "feisti-ness," as actress and breast cancer survivor Suzanne Somers once described it. You see it everywhere.

The most fundamental and empowering belief is that cancer does not mean death.

Survivors come to grips with this truth: cancer may or may not mean death. This set of beliefs, attitudes, and resulting emotions carries a vastly different outlook from either the superpositive or the hopelessly negative patients. "Yes, I may die," said Chris, a thirty-something California housewife. "But I also may live. In fact, I am going to live to the fullest. I am not going to die of fear and hopelessness."

That attitude correlates with survivorship. The beliefs extend to medical treatments and potential side effects. Survivors tend to envision their treatments as highly effective. They further believe side effects will be minimal and manageable. The 50 Essential Things You Can Do detailed in chapter 7 will help you understand and apply these attitudes of healing to your own core recovery program.

You will not be surprised to learn survivors believe they have the absolute central role in the recovery process. This belief and resulting attitude is at complete odds with millions of other cancer patients who defer virtually every question to their doctors. Not survivors.

It's surprising: survivors have a love/hate relationship with their medical team. They want the best of care and respect those healthcare professionals who speak truth and patiently explain what evidence supports their treatment recommendations and what out-comes can be expected. But if that information is not freely forth-coming, survivors can be exceptionally confrontational. Survivors check and recheck physician recommendations, often challenging tests, treatments, and prognoses. Many survivors change doctors in search of those in whom they have the most trust.

#5 Support

Survivors invest time and emotional energy in relationships that nurture them. They also invest less time and energy in relationships that are toxic. While this may seem to be a benign practice, it has some surprising health implications that survivors consider important.

Loving relationships with friends, relatives, lovers, spouses, children, coworkers and employees—or the lack of those relationships—build us up or tear us down. Survivors tend to become "relationship sensitive," examining, perhaps for the first time in their lives, how they get along with other people.

Survivors seem to be able to grasp the high value of now—the simple and readily available life that is theirs in spite of cancer.

It is quite common for survivors to put difficult relationships on hold, especially during any debilitating treatments. This does not mean survivors exile toxic people from their lives for all time. But it certainly signals reduced emotional investment in those relationships.

Breast cancer tends to give patients the permission to examine a wide variety of life choices, especially their network of social support. They often make changes. I personally worked with Tina, a breast cancer patient who had long-standing difficulty in her relationship with her mother. "I was always being criticized. And during treatment, I needed encouragement. So I told her no more visits or phone calls until I called her. It was over three months before I contacted her. But I needed room to focus on healing."

Tina's example is very helpful because much of the work of getting well again takes place within one's social support network. The last thing a breast cancer patient needs is a toxic person second-guessing and criticizing every decision.

New and important research is now demonstrating the health benefits of supportive relationships. Survivors have at least one person with whom they can share anything—everything—without fear of judgment or condemnation. That is a powerful healing elixir.

#6 Spiritual

Cancer survivors embrace a more spiritual perspective. They repeatedly speak of seeing life differently now compared with prior to their diagnosis and treatment. This spiritual outlook stands in marked contrast to other cancer patients who obsess over a body that may be riddled with disease or who mourn endlessly over dreams that are hopelessly derailed. Survivors seem to be able to grasp the high value of now—the simple and readily available life that is theirs in spite of cancer.

This more spiritual perspective is not an issue of religion. Many survivors reject traditional religious practices. It's the old adage: just because you sit in a garage does not mean you will become a car, and just because you sit in a church or synagogue does not mean you will become more spiritual. And clearly, no single doctrine or creed brings prepackaged answers to all.

Nor does this spirituality simply consist of bland platitudes. Instead, the transformation is typically seen as an inner peace, a serenity, a quiet confidence, a more grateful and joyful way of living. In a very real sense, they have come to let God work in and through them. Celeste, a breast cancer survivor, explained the essential nature of the spiritual walk. She said, "Now, when I walk into a room, I am there serving as God's representative." For millions of cancer survivors, this is the apex of the healing journey.

Implementation Intelligence

This is our framework for recovery. Each of these six strategies is important, even essential, to breast cancer survival. However, they are not always equal. Timing is one issue. If the decision is made to consider and commence a recommended medical treatment, nearly all the emphasis is on that area. Once in place, survivors tend to let the doctors treat while they move on to implement programs that include nutrition, exercise, attitude, and the range of holistic aspects of getting well again.

Implementation of one principle typically follows another at the appropriate time. Few survivors make simultaneous wholesale changes. Those who do attempt to change too much too quickly often meet with temporary defeat and have to start again.

Each principle has its important place in survival. Many breast cancer survivors note that solving a relationship issue may have been just as important in their recovery as medical treatment. Adopting a healthy nutritional program and making a commitment to daily exercise may be on par with the contribution of radiation or chemotherapy.

It takes us back to where we started. Once again, I ask you to view your state of health as a result of the many interactive components of body, mind, and spirit. Cell biology may be one component, but overall health is more often the result of our lifestyle choices.

Breast cancer recovery becomes a healing symphony. The survivors believe they have earned their return to health, aligning themselves with their own immense healing capacity. "The music of my healing springs from within," said Brandi. "I simply had to release it."

So let's summarize to this point. The integration of these six key strategies creates the framework for patients to follow in the breast cancer recovery journey:

Medicine	Attitude
Nutrition	Support
Exercise	Spirituality

The cancer survival pyramid is the context, the strategic plan, in which the 50 Essential Things You Can Do are implemented. It's your road map. Consult it often.

❦ 7 ❧
The 50 Essential
Things You Can Do

The First Step on the Incredible Journey: Understand Your Diagnosis

Your number one priority following a cancer diagnosis is to put in place the best integrated cancer care program you can possibly design. To do so, you must first understand your diagnosis. And this is much more than simply going to one doctor and saying, "Treat me."

The decisions you make regarding your cancer care and recovery program are some of the most important you will make in your entire life. I encourage you to begin the journey through breast cancer by following this course of action that has proven highly effective for tens of thousands of survivors.

#1

Focus

You've been told, "It's cancer." I have deep compassion for you. I can appreciate your feelings. I've been there, too.

First, you're in shock and filled with fear. The next moment you're angry but not quite certain at what or whom. Then come the thoughts of "How did this happen? Why me?" Even the guilt starts to creep in: "Did I bring this on myself?" Plus, all the questions have started to rush through your mind: "Will I die? How long do I have? What will happen to my family?" And on and on and on. Your mind is overwhelmed at times.

Stop. Be calm. Try not to panic. Focus. Yes, I know that this is easier said than done.

Breast cancer is a serious illness. But let's be clear: breast cancer is not necessarily fatal. In fact, if your cancer is contained in the breast, the chances are excellent that you will be among the nine in ten women who survive at least five years and hopefully more.

You do have the luxury of at least some time. Unlike a severed artery, cancer does not require you to do something this very instant.

A hurried response, based in fear and panic, is neither required nor preferred. A hurried response may be harmful. However, please don't take that as a license for inaction.

A hurried response, based in fear and panic, is neither required nor preferred. A hurried response may be harmful. However, please don't take that as a license for inaction.

Stop and examine your frenzied thoughts for just a moment. It is at the beginning stages of this journey that clear decision making will be most important. With your early decisions, you will ensure that your illness is properly treated. Panic acts only to your detriment.

Panic is a mental phenomenon, a response to our thoughts about cancer being frightful and overpowering. The process can accurately be labeled as "awfulizing." Isn't that an apt description? When we awfulize, we take our current situation to its worst possible conclusion.

If we will observe our emotions objectively for just a moment, we will see something different from initial appearances. The intense panic that virtually every breast cancer patient initially experiences is actually the mind projecting its fears about the unknown future. Think about it and understand this truth: Panic is caused by an assumption based in fear. It is not based on material fact.

What to do when you start to feel anxious emotions arising inside? Try to witness them. Just observe. You may want to give those emotions an image. View them, and yourself, in your mind's eye. Instead of putting yourself in the role of a victim who is hopelessly caught in a web of panic and despair, become the observer. By not engaging the mind in battle, by simply watching the emotions and letting go, your panic will soon subside.

Then imagine yourself as an effective problem solver. Give yourself an image of a competent and confident person who is about to make some very important choices. Clear decision making can and will be yours.

An Essential Thing You Can Do

Sit down. Take a deep breath. Say out loud, "Cancer does not mean death." Observe your emotions. Detach by separating who you are as a person from the emotional panic you may be feeling. You are not uncontrolled panic, even though you may be experiencing panic. Understand that difference. Now immediately read and act on steps #2 and #3.

#2
Put Yourself in Charge

Who is the most important person on your breast cancer recovery team? Some people believe it is their surgeon. Others believe it is their oncologist. Some choose the medical technicians, others the nurse, and still others choose their spouse.

But the most important person on your health and healing team is you! You are the one who is ill. It is you who must work to get well again. You are the character of central importance. You are in charge.

Much too often, patients surrender leadership. Anita, a fifty-two-year-old woman from Iowa, was diagnosed with metastatic breast cancer. Her treatment was not progressing as expected, and the side effects depleted her. It all left Anita understandably discouraged. Her doctor kept assuring her, "We're doing all we can. Trust me."

Following an especially difficult week, Anita considered her options. "Do I accept the course of this treatment or do I try something new? I called and made an appointment at a Mayo Clinic's Comprehensive Cancer Center. It was a four-hour drive from my home." Doctors there recommended a different treatment program that Anita took back to her home doctor for implementation. "Personally taking charge was my turning point," explained a healthy Anita four years after her bold and assertive decision.

It is you who must work to get well again. You are the character of central importance. You are in charge.

Survivors take charge. View yourself as the owner of a fashionable restaurant, or whatever organizational analogy you like. This is your cancer recovery organization, and the mission is to get you well again. You'll want a strong general manager; many times that is your family doctor or perhaps a naturopath. And you'll need other team members: a chef, a prep chef, waiters, bus staff, and a smiling greeter to welcome your customers. Equate all these with specialists: your surgeon, medical oncologist, radiation oncologist, nutritionist, and more. You, the restaurant owner, interview the candidates and employ your staff. You make the decisions.

Taking charge is a significant step for many patients. Traditionally, consumers play a passive role in the healthcare system, going along with virtually whatever doctors and allied health care professionals recommend. We're encouraged to consent to rather than to challenge recommendations. This passive attitude does not serve you well.

An Essential Thing You Can Do

Evaluate your team. Who are the players? Who is managing this team? Is it a one-person show? How many more people could be helping? Are the team members working for you, or do some seem to be working against you? One woman remarked, "Every time I go to the doctor, I feel like I am in enemy territory." If you feel that way, it's time to make a change. Take charge!

3

Ask Your Doctor These Questions

It is critically important for you to clearly understand your diagnosis and the proposed treatment. The doctor who diagnosed you should answer the following questions. Transcribe these questions and record the answers in your Wellness and Recovery Journal:

1. Precisely what type of cancer do I have?

2. Has the cancer spread beyond the primary site? If so, where?

3. What tests did you use to determine this diagnosis?

4. Is there any indication that a second pathology report is needed?

5. Are you recommending additional tests? What are you looking for with each test?

6. How certain are you that the tests and the resulting diagnosis are accurate?

7. What are my treatment options? Which one(s) do you recommend? (Record these recommendations in precise detail.)

8. Whom would you recommend for a second opinion?

9. Are you a board-certified oncologist?

10. Will you put me in touch with patients whom you have successfully treated?

As a cancer patient, you are a consumer. The decision process regarding who will prescribe and administer your treatment is not that much different from any other major purchase decision. But the consequences of your decisions are radically different from those involved in buying a refrigerator, for example.

You have the right and the responsibility to ask questions of your doctor just as you would with any consumer purchase. Evaluate those answers more closely than questions you may have asked for any major purchase you have ever made. Your options and choices for the best treatment will then become clear.

Breast cancer survivors are consumer activists. They ask. Become an activist!

An Essential Thing You Can Do

Obtain answers to the preceding questions today! Record the answers in your Wellness and Recovery Journal. Ask the same questions once again at the time you obtain your second opinion.

#4

Obtain a Second Opinion

Obtain a second opinion from a board-certified oncologist, a cancer specialist. This is a critically important step that is not to be overlooked. If at all possible, the second opinion should be completed prior to starting any treatment program.

Whom you consult is also critically important. The second opinion should come from an independent oncologist who is not in a working partnership, formal or informal, with the doctor who made the initial diagnosis. If possible, the second opinion should be given by an oncologist who is in a different medical group from the first. Yes, you're looking for a truly independent second opinion.

You are also looking for a multidisciplinary second opinion. Do you recall our discussion regarding the hammer syndrome? This revealed that medical specialists tend to recommend their specialty. Surgeons see treatment as surgery. Radiation oncologists want to employ radiation. Medical oncologists see breast cancer through the lens of pharmaceutical treatments.

You seek to understand all your treatment options based on all these medical disciplines—and more. You are most likely to obtain a multidisciplinary second opinion at a major cancer center. I encourage you to find such a center, especially if the diagnosis indicates a more advanced cancer, Stage III or IV.

Yes, it's more work. Yes, there is more expense. But please assert yourself and obtain a second opinion. This part of your breast cancer journey is absolutely crucial. Please take this guidance literally.

I do understand that requesting a second opinion may appear daunting to many patients. Do not be fearful that a request for a second opinion might alienate your doctor. Second-opinion consultations are standard procedure. Your oncologist makes such referrals every day.

Ask the doctor or a member of the staff who made the initial diagnosis for a complete transcript of your medical records. There may be a small charge for these records, and it may take a day or two. Then bring the records to your second-opinion doctor or have them sent ahead. I prefer to personally hand the records to the consulting staff. It eliminates the chance of lost records and delays.

In the United States, the cost of obtaining at least one second opinion is reimbursed by virtually all insurance programs. Even if you're not covered, get a second opinion. Don't let cost stand in the way of obtaining some of the most important advice of your life.

"I had a second opinion all right," explained Katherine, a fifty-five-year-old insurance office manager and grandmother, describing her experience with breast cancer. "The second opinion came from another surgeon who shared offices with the first. They both said that a radical [mastectomy] was the way to go. And to this day I wonder if I would have been better off with a lumpectomy."

Katherine's second-opinion experience could have been improved in two ways. First, she would have been better served by consulting with an oncologist. These specialists diagnose and treat cancer every working day. They can and should be expected to have up-to-date information on treatment options for each type and stage of cancer. Both surgeons Katherine consulted were general surgeons who dealt with a variety of illnesses, not just cancer.

Second, Katherine would have been better served by consulting with a second-opinion doctor not associated with the first. Her surgeons were located in the same building and just down the hall from her family doctor.

These associations are a little-discussed but potentially important issue to patients. Doctors who are friends, officemates, business associates, or in a junior position within a medical practice may find it difficult to challenge the diagnoses or recommended treatment programs of associates. All sorts of relationships exist that may influence decisions.

Years ago, we uncovered a troubling situation in Orange County, California. Second-opinion referrals were routinely being made from one community-based oncologist to another. The second oncologist would reciprocate. Both were well-known and had very large practices. Patients would come to our support group and share. It quickly became apparent that the first and second opinions always concurred. It seemed obvious that the two doctors simply agreed with each other's treatment recommendations. We stopped making referrals to both.

That experience may seem improbable, but unfortunately the story is true. The best safeguard is to seek a second opinion from a board-certified oncologist who is affiliated with a different practice, works in a different hospital, perhaps even lives in a different city than the doctor making the initial diagnosis. Cancer centers endorsed by the National Cancer Institute are the gold standard for conventionally based second-opinion consultations. You can find the one nearest you at *http://cancercenters.cancer.gov/cancer_centers/*.

I want to encourage you to gently confront any fears you may have about asking for a second opinion. I know that the typical thought process about second opinions includes "Well, I don't want to offend my doctor."

Obtaining a second opinion in no way implies that the initial diagnosis is incorrect or that the suggested treatment is inappropriate. On a subject as important as this, you simply deserve to have the benefit of more than one person's thinking. Your second opinion search also puts you in touch with other doctors, giving you options and helping you decide which medical team will actually administer your treatment program.

Obtaining a second opinion in no way implies that the initial diagnosis is incorrect or that the suggested treatment is inappropriate.

An Essential Thing You Can Do

Make your appointment for a second opinion today. This is one of the most important things you can do. *Do not overlook this step.* Act now! Pick up the phone. Make the appointment.

5

Become an e-Patient

You can turn to the Internet to help you through the breast cancer journey. Here you can more fully research your diagnosis, understand the details of all your treatment options, and even connect with other patients similarly diagnosed. Here is a handful of the best resources:

Breast Cancer Charities of America
www.thebreastcancercharities.org

> The award-winning resource for integrated cancer care, the Breast Cancer Charities of America site helps you mobilize body, mind, and spirit to get well and stay well. Here you will also find an important analysis of conventional, complementary, and alternative treatment options. Also provided are extensive nutritional guidance, exercise options, and attitude builders. Here you can also be directed to both individual and group support, online and via telephone. Spiritually inclusive.

National Cancer Institute
www.cancer.gov/cancertopics/types/breast

> If you need more technical and medically focused information, this is your source. Extensive information is available here on breast cancer statistics, diagnosis, conventional treatment options, genetics, clinical trials, and ongoing research.

BreastCancer.org
www.breastcancer.org

> BreastCancer.org is an excellent medically oriented site communicating in nonmedical language. It includes information on symptoms and diagnosis, treatment, and side effects, and it hosts chatrooms in which you can connect with other patients.

There is a plethora of breast cancer information on the web. I encourage you to spend time here obtaining answers to your questions on diagnosis and treatment. Even more important, use the Internet to understand how you can create health and healing—how you can get well and stay well.

Use the Internet to understand how you can create health and healing—how you can get well and stay well.

An Essential Thing You Can Do

Do the research. Hold yourself accountable for gaining a working knowledge of your diagnosis and all your treatment options.

#6

Reframe the Statistics

As you conduct the research into your conventional, complementary, and alternative treatment options, you will invariably discover cancer recovery statistics that detail cancer incidence, mortality, and five-year survival rates. Do not let these statistics paralyze you.

Statistics measure populations. They can be interpreted in a great many ways. But statistics do not determine any individual case, including yours.

Let's look squarely at the facts about breast cancer. According to the National Cancer Institute and the Centers of Disease Control and Prevention, here's what the numbers tell us:

The starting point: Nine in ten women who are diagnosed with breast cancer will survive at least five years. Five years out from diagnosis is the standard "you are cured" milestone. Yes, we need to do better, and there is much room for improvement. But look at your own situation and think, "I have a 90 percent chance of survival." That's good.

About one in eight women in the United States will develop invasive breast cancer over the course of her lifetime. In 2010, an estimated 207,000 new cases of invasive breast cancer were diagnosed along with 54,000 new cases of noninvasive (in situ) breast cancer. In addition, about 2,000 new cases of invasive breast cancer were diagnosed in men. Note that less than 1 percent of all new breast cancer cases occur in men.

From 1999 to 2006, breast cancer incidence rates in the United States decreased by about 2 percent per year. This decrease is correlated most closely with the reduced use of hormone replacement therapy (HRT) by women. HRT increased the incidence of breast cancer. Understand this point: the decrease in incidence was due to ceasing the use of conventional medicine, not adding more medicine. As you know by now, this recurring theme of less is more is the foundation of this book.

About forty thousand women in the United States died in 2010 from breast cancer. Death rates have been decreasing since 1991. The good news is that there are now more than 2.5 million breast cancer survivors in the United States.

Compared to African American women, white women are slightly more likely to develop breast cancer but less likely to die of it. One possible reason is that African American women tend to have more aggressive tumors, although why this is the case is not known. Women of other ethnic backgrounds—Asian, Hispanic, and Native American—have a lower risk of developing and dying from breast cancer than either whites or African Americans.

A woman's risk of breast cancer approximately doubles if she has a first-degree relative (mother, sister, daughter) who has been diagnosed with breast cancer. About 25 percent of women diagnosed with breast cancer have a family history of breast cancer. Approximately 5 to 10 percent of breast cancers can be linked to gene mutations (abnormal changes) inherited from one's mother or father. Mutations of the BRCA1 and 2 genes are the most common. Women with these mutations have up to an 80 percent risk of developing breast cancer during their lifetime, and they are more likely to be diagnosed at a younger age, before menopause. An increased ovarian cancer risk is also associated with these genetic mutations.

There is no type of breast cancer that does not have some rate of survival. This is a significant fact. It is also cause for reasonable hope.

This means that approximately 75 percent of breast cancers occur in women who have no family history of the disease. It is thought these cancers occur due to genetic abnormalities that happen as a result of the aging process and life in general, rather than from inherited mutations. The most significant risk factors for breast cancer are gender, (being a woman) and age (growing older).

No matter how difficult your diagnosis, even if it's a recurrence, please realize that there is no type of breast cancer that does not have some rate of survival. This is a significant fact. It is also cause for reasonable hope. The question now becomes, "What can I do to maximize my chances of getting on the right side of these statistics?"

An Essential Thing You Can Do

Reframe the statistics. Interpret them as indications of progress. Determine to act with the conviction that hope is your greatest ally and that you will do all within your power to be counted among the survivor statistics.

The Second Step on the Incredible Journey:
Plan Your Treatment

Breast cancer calls for a rational plan of treatment. And after understanding your diagnosis, you will have several options to consider. Much of the conventional treatment recommendations will depend on a combination of your pathology report and the treatment customs in your geographic area.

You have the central role to play in this decision. And your treatment plan needs to balance the physician's recommendations with your wishes. You are in charge. This section will help you make a step-by-step evaluation to arrive at the treatment plan that is right for you. So let's move on to this next series of decisions.

#7

Understand Your Conventional
Treatment Options

Let's again briefly summarize your conventional breast cancer treatment options. You can expect treatment recommendations to fall into one or a combination of three primary treatment modalities:

- Surgery: removal of the tumor
- Radiation: exposure to X-rays or radium
- Chemotherapy: the use of cytotoxic chemicals

Surgery is the most frequently employed breast cancer treatment. It is best used when the cancer is small and has not moved to other parts of the body.

Radiation therapy is employed in approximately half of all breast cancer cases. It is often used in combination with other treatment options, for example after lumpectomy.

Chemotherapy is most often used when the cancer has spread or when it is thought the tumor needs to be reduced in size prior to surgery. Chemotherapy is often used in combination with radiation therapy and surgery in an attempt to prevent recurrence or control tumor growth.

Three other types of conventional medical treatments are:

- Hormonal: manipulation of your body's natural hormones
- Immunotherapy: enhancement of the body's own immune function
- Investigative: experimental programs

Hormonal treatment is used in breast cancers that depend on hormones such as estrogen and progesterone for their growth. Hormones are either removed or added, or their production is blocked through drugs. Cancer that is hormone sensitive is slower growing and typically responds to hormone-suppression treatment. Hormone-negative cancer does not call for this kind of treatment. To be sure, there are pharmaceuticals that seek to mitigate this condition. The most prominent hormone-suppressing drugs are tamoxifen and raloxifene, often employed as a follow-up in an attempt to prevent recurrence.

Immunotherapies are an attempt to boost or restore the body's natural defense system. Many people believe immunotherapies will soon comprise a fourth widely accepted treatment modality.

Human epidermal growth factor 2–positive (HER2-positive) breast cancer is one type of breast cancer. This is characterized by aggressive growth and typically linked with a poor prognosis. Approximately one in five breast cancers are HER2 positive. While HER2 refers to a genetic condition, the problem is not inherited but more likely the result of aging and a less-than-healthful lifestyle. You can expect testing will be done to determine your HER2 status. While research is early, there is compelling evidence that HER2 overexpression is one of those classic cases where improved lifestyle is able to stop the expression.

Not surprisingly, there are drugs for HER2-positive breast cancer patients, such as Herceptin and Tykerb. They are targeted immunotherapies and most often used in conjunction with other drugs. A long list of side effects can be viewed at *www.drugwatch.com.*

Investigative protocols are experimental. They are typically the last choice.

As you evaluate your conventional treatment options, please consider some of my personal observations from over a quarter century of helping patients make informed choices:

1. Surgery is the most common form of conventional treatment for breast cancer. It is also the most effective. Unless you are at Stage 0 or Stage IV, I urge you to consider the surgery. Generally, the only choices are mastectomy versus lumpectomy, lymph node removal versus sentinel lymph node dissection.

2. If you agree to surgery, the decision as to who actually performs the procedure is yours. Your choice of surgeons is important.

You're more likely to get a well-qualified surgeon if you choose one who is a fellow of the American College of Surgeons and who is also board certified in his or her field. Only about half of practicing surgeons are board certified, so be sure to ask.

Special note to premenopausal breast cancer patients:

You typically have some flexibility on the timing of your surgery. As we previously noted, scientific evidence is mounting that fewer breast cancer recurrences are reported among women who choose to have their surgery during the luteal, or latter, phase of the menstrual cycle, i.e., fourteen to thirty days following the onset of menstruation. Except for one Canadian study which suggested the eighth day after menstruation onset to be the optimal time, research shows surgery performed in the latter half of the menstrual cycle results in the fewest recurrences. You may have to assert yourself here; most surgeries are scheduled at the convenience of the surgeon and/or the hospital.

3. Thoroughly understand chemotherapy. Before you say yes to chemotherapy, ask to see proof, such as scientific papers and reports, on the effectiveness of the treatment being offered. Examine the hard evidence that the suggested chemotherapy protocol actually cures, extends life, or improves quality of life. Those are the three outcomes against which you must measure all treatments—conventional, experimental, complementary, or alternative.

   If your clinician uses the terms *response* or *tumor response*, *surrogate markers* or *reduce the tumor burden*, these represent different standards. These terms mean shrinkage and a corresponding reduction in the immune-suppressive effect the tumor has. None of these terms is synonymous with *cure*.

   The word *cure* must be used very carefully in breast cancer. In fact, if you find a clinician who uses the word loosely, in the context that he can guarantee a cure, don't walk away—run! You deserve someone with more credibility.

A cure actually requires that your immune system eventually successfully keeps the cancer in check. Cure is more than treatment and indicates that your immune system can maintain a disease-free state. To maximize your opportunity for such a response, I encourage you to follow as many of the health-enhancing, life-enriching principles in this book as possible.

Study the chemotherapy treatment option in depth. Do your own research. Ask about both short-term and long-term side effects. Request the names and phone numbers of long-term survivors who were treated with similar regimens. Ask them to share their experience. Know exactly what you can expect—and not expect—this recommended treatment option to accomplish. Once you possess that information, you are in a position to make a truly informed decision.

4. The administration of chemotherapy is not an exact science. Ask your oncologist about chemotherapy sensitivity (in vitro) testing. Here, samples of your tissue are chemically analyzed in laboratory tests to determine interaction with different agents. In about a week, your oncologist will receive a report establishing which drugs are not likely to work as well as the most active agents. The net effect is hopefully a personalized treatment program optimized before you begin.

5. Chemotherapy may be in pill form, to be taken orally, or it may be in liquid form and injected into a muscle. But most commonly, chemo is given through a vein. The drugs may be administered in a daily, weekly, or monthly program for periods ranging from a few months to a lifetime. Side effects, once the fear of all patients, are now being more effectively controlled and vary widely from individual to individual. Refer to "#14 Overcome Fatigue and Nausea," in the next section for helpful actions you can take to control uncomfortable side effects.

6. Radiation therapy is most often administered by means of an external beam machine. Internal radiation is becoming more common, where radioactive seeds are surgically implanted into

or on the area to be treated. This procedure requires precision. You will maximize your opportunity for receiving excellent care if you choose a physician who is certified by the American Board of Radiology. Ask.

All breast cancers are treatable. Even in cases where the cancer is advanced, experimental investigative programs are available. If your cancer is not responding to conventional treatment, ask about hormonal treatment and biological response modifiers. Especially consider the many complementary and alternative programs described in this book. You are entitled to understand the full range of treatments available. From that understanding, you will have the knowledge and power to make the most intelligent treatment decisions.

Once again, conventional treatment has its important place. In interviews with thousands of cancer survivors, over 96 percent stated they initiated a course of conventional therapy. As much as I am exceedingly concerned about the probability that you may be overdiagnosed and overtreated, it is incorrect to report that cancer survivors turn exclusively to alternative, nontraditional cancer treatments.

In the late 1980s, a Food and Drug Administration study estimated that 40 percent of cancer patients use nontraditional treatments. I believe the number may now be much higher, perhaps 70 to 80 percent. But clearly, survivors do not give up the traditional treatments. They integrate complementary and alternative practices into a comprehensive recovery program. Breast cancer survivors go beyond treating the illness; they create health and healing. That is what this guidance is all about. I ask you to do the same.

An Essential Thing You Can Do

Ask your oncologist to explain the specific treatment options available to you in the areas of surgery, radiation, and chemotherapy. Ask also about hormonal, immunotherapy, and investigative programs.

Ask for his or her recommendation. Record this information in your Wellness and Recovery Journal. *Do not give your approval for treatment just yet. First, more work remains to be completed.*

#8

Gauge Your Confidence in Your Medical Team

Few patients have any objective way to judge whether their surgeons, oncologists, or other medical professionals have high-level technical competence. We can consider our medical team's education and professional certifications and the experiences of other patients. But few of us can evaluate, with technical accuracy, whether a particular doctor will be able to address our specific case with success. We can, however, make subjective assessments, the kind of judgments that can be enormously important in our recovery journey. We can intuitively gauge our confidence level.

Malcolm Gladwell, in his intriguing book *Blink*, explores the ideas around the choices that we make in an instant. He especially explores the idea of our "intuitive repulsion," where in as little as a few seconds, we are able to understand more about the essence of a person—often in a single glance—than through weeks or months of analysis. This same idea applies to our confidence in our medical team. And it relates directly to the power of the mind-body connection.

It may seem strange that after encouraging you to carefully do your homework and analyze your treatment options that I now raise the idea of a more intuitive judgment. But here is what is strange and true. Cancer patients who do well not only have confidence in their doctors, they esteem their doctors.

Cancer patients who do well not only have confidence in their doctors, they esteem their doctors.

In more than twenty-five years of this work, we have noted that the phenomenon of the doctor-patient relationship is consistently profound. And we have observed that the relationship precedes rather than follows the health outcome. There seems to be a direct correlation: Positive relationship equals positive treatment outcome. Negative relationship equals negative, or at least less successful, outcome.

The phenomenon seems to be related to how patients are treated, on a personal level, by their doctors. Remember Ruth, the family physician diagnosed with breast cancer. Her relationship with her colleague the surgeon changed once Ruth was in the role of patient. Ruth shared that his professional manner became rushed, her questions were dismissed, and she was treated poorly.

In our telesupport group work, we take note of the literally thousands of patients who have complained about their doctors and shared their own version of intuitive repulsion. More times than we can count, we have heard "I hate my doctor," or "He never takes time to really talk to me," or "He sees me as a breast cancer, not as a whole person."

Supportive doctor/patient relationships are to be expected by every patient. Look for behavior in the examination room that helps you understand the process. This could be statements like "At today's appointment, I want to review the results of the tests, conduct another clinical breast examination, and then discuss our treatment options," or "Let me share with you what the biopsy report is telling us, and then I'll review the steps of a lumpectomy."

Look for the tone of voice from your medical team that communicates compassion and concern, not dominance and superiority. In the end, you are looking for a doctor who shows you respect and unconditional regard.

Your intuition about your caretakers is important. Look for the tone of voice from your medical team that communicates compassion and concern, not dominance and superiority. In the end, you are looking for a doctor who shows you respect and unconditional regard.

I believe that confidence in your medical team, or lack of confidence, directly correlates with outcome. I believe you can trust your intuition, provided you double-check it. To be sure, an excellent bedside manner can seldom make up for a lack of training, knowledge, and technical competence. But survivors have repeatedly told me there is a direct correlation between the confidence one has in one's healthcare team and one's probability of recovery.

An Essential Thing You Can Do

The next time you meet with your doctor, analyze his tone of voice and his level of respect for you and especially determine if he is asking you questions and listening to your responses. Evaluate your confidence level following that encounter. If he is talking down to you or isn't listening to you, or if you feel he isn't treating you with respect, listen to your intuition. This is particularly important when you are being asked to make treatment decisions. If you harbor more doubt than assurance toward your healthcare providers and their treatment recommendations, it is time to change either your confidence level or your team.

. . . .

Take a Break

Be sure you are approaching this work at a comfortable pace. I suggest you take a break now and reflect on this important step. Continue your work after you have rested.

#9

Seek Conviction versus Wishful Thinking

As I write this, we are currently counseling Joan, a fifty-three-year-old wife and a mother of two college-age girls. Joan is also an elementary school teacher. Earlier this year, in the middle of Joan's hectic schedule, came a suspicious mammogram. She was told she would need to discuss this with her primary care doctor as soon as possible.

Joan is exceedingly adverse to invasive diagnosis techniques and toxic treatments. After her doctor explained the situation and her options, Joan asked for an ultrasound. Depending on those results, decisions could be made if further tests were required or treatment needed to be considered.

The ultrasound came back positive. This was more than just a cyst or minor calcification. Her primary care physician suggested that this be treated as if it were malignant. The recommendation: a lumpectomy to remove the suspicious lump and a small amount of the surrounding tissue. Joan balked. She didn't like the idea of surgery—any kind of surgery. This seemed way too radical. Instead, she agreed to an MRI (magnetic resonance imaging) and a BRCA gene test.

Even though it took nearly six weeks to schedule the MRI, the test results finally came back. The BRCA test showed she carried the genetic mutation, and the MRI showed several suspicious areas. Again, lumpectomy was recommended. And again, Joan refused. Instead she agreed to a fine needle biopsy. The results were definitive. This was IBC, inflammatory breast cancer, and the MRI readings indicated that it was probably Stage III.

Joan still resisted surgery. Instead, she agreed to a series of six chemotherapy treatments consisting of Taxotere, Carboplatin, and Herceptin. Now, just as she is finishing the last of her six treatments, the tests show the tumors to be smaller but still present. The recommendation: mastectomy with removal of the axillary lymph nodes.

Joan called us in a panic: "I hate the thought of surgery. One of my teacher colleagues had surgery, and it was botched. She contracted sepsis and eventually died." She added, "I thought the chemo would be enough."

Of course we are counseling surgery. At this hour, Joan remains uncertain as to the correct course of action.

We also recommended Joan search out nontraditional treatments. We put her in touch with a naturopath who suggested metabolic therapy, a combination of detoxification, herbs, and hyperthermia—the use of heat—to help destroy cancer cells. While this program seems minimally toxic and noninvasive, Joan has now expressed the fear she was getting too far away from conventional medical care.

How Joan's case will be resolved is not clear. And her resistance to surgery is clearly not the answer for everyone. But following one's conviction is an important element of nearly every successful treatment program.

An Essential Thing You Can Do

Before you commit to a treatment program, take the time to ask some critical questions: "Do I hold the belief that this is the right thing to be doing, or am I just taking the path of least resistance?" If you don't believe in it, resist! Find a treatment program that you can follow with conviction.

#10
Reflect on the Treatment Decision

If you've carefully read each step up to this point, you'll realize that you've simply been gathering information about your breast cancer treatment options. You have not yet made any treatment decisions. Now it is time to systematically review your treatment options one last time prior to crossing this Rubicon.

First, compare. Are you receiving consistent information from:

- The doctor who made the initial diagnosis
- The oncologist whom you consulted for your second opinion
- The recommendations you found through your independent research

You should expect to see a reasonable consistency in the recommendations you receive from these sources. Most treatment variances should relate to differences in levels of toxicity and degrees of invasiveness. If there is fundamental agreement, your decision-making process will probably be straightforward.

If the recommendations are inconsistent, then your information gathering is not complete. When you receive mixed signals, it is a certain sign to obtain a third qualified and independent opinion. This is time and money wisely spent.

Several prominent professionals in the oncology community have criticized me for this suggestion. They have expressed contrary recommendations to their patients such as "The differences in treatment that you'll find are actually very minor," and "You're just losing valuable time in receiving treatment."

I disagree.

In all but the very rare case, several days spent in gaining a third or fourth opinion

> *When you receive mixed signals, it is a certain sign to obtain a third qualified and independent opinion. This is time and money wisely spent.*

are well worth the wait. As a patient, you seek the very best treatment. You should expect a consistency of recommendations, if not a consensus.

We worked with a woman who lived in a rural part of a Southern state. Between her family physician, a report from a mobile mammography test, and a follow-up visit at a university-based cancer center, she received three different recommendations. We encouraged her to look further, even to the point of paying for another appointment because she did not have adequate health insurance.

Once you attain clarity and conviction in terms of the medical treatment, another evaluation needs a second reflective look. Are you comfortable with the people who will give you treatment and the place where the treatment will be administered?

We recently helped a woman change doctors because she literally could not understand the resident physician. She said, "I know this sounds as if I am wantonly prejudiced, but his English was so poor that I could not put my life into the hands of a young resident from some foreign country whom I could not understand." If you experience something similar, do the same.

Even a change of facilities is appropriate. Toni underwent surgery at a major cancer center on the west side of Los Angeles. However, she lived in Riverside, a suburb on the far eastern edge of the Los Angeles metropolitan area. Depending on traffic, the commute was an hour or more one way. When they attempted to schedule her for radiation, five days a week for seven weeks, Toni said, "No. I can't stand that commute." She found a radiation oncologist within twenty minutes of her home. If you experience something similar, do the same.

Does the recommended treatment program truly have your conviction? Are you convinced the people and even the place where you will be treated are the best? Conviction implies a sense of certainty. While there are no guarantees, your treatment program, as well as the people who administer it, should elicit a strong degree of certainty that this is the right path to be taking at this time.

One more point. In analyzing treatment options, invariably the question arises, "What about all the alternative approaches? I really haven't checked them out." We have consistently recommended this strategy: First, explore the conventional treatment options. Surgery, radiation, and chemotherapy are the basis for the overwhelming majority of survivor success stories. If the conventional treatment methods hold no real promise, and particularly if they are unsuccessful, then analyze the complementary and alternative therapies. With all the options, integrate improved diet, exercise, nutritional supplementation, plus the psychosocial and psychospiritual techniques.

Allow yourself time to reflect on these important decisions. Don't be pressured by anyone to make a quick decision. When the treatment recommendations are consistent, the people who administer the treatment have your confidence; you understand the importance of integrating body, mind, and spirit; and you can say with conviction that this is what you should be doing. Then, and only then, are you ready to go to the next step.

An Essential Thing You Can Do

Consult your notations in your Wellness and Recovery Journal. Thoughtfully, carefully, systematically, reflect on your treatment decision.

. . . .

Take a Break

Take another break. Reflect . . . again.

#11

Decide!

There is power in decision.

The breast cancer journey is made up of both little decisions and big decisions. Your treatment program is a big decision. In many ways it will determine the direction of your entire life. Now is the time to decide.

Decision is the spark that ignites action. Until a decision is reached, nothing happens.

Making decisions like this takes courage. But there is power in facing the fact that you have breast cancer, then carefully doing your homework, and finally choosing a course of action. Without exercising your courage, the problem will remain forever unaddressed.

Decide! Don't straddle the fence or make a partial decision. This is the time to take a firm stand on one side or another. Make a full commitment.

Yes, you will monitor your decision. You will keep your options open, of course. But now is the moment to say, "This is how we will climb the mountain! Now let's get started!"

Decision frees us from many of the uncertainties caused by fear, doubt, and anxiety. Yes, there is risk. But there is greater risk in making no decision, hoping that all will magically be well.

> *Decision frees us from many of the uncertainties caused by fear, doubt, and anxiety. Yes, there is risk. But there is greater risk in making no decision, hoping that all will magically be well.*

Decide. You've done the work. You've balanced that against your intuition. This is not blind chance. This decision is the culmination of careful and sustained inquiry. Now is the time for action.

Decision awakens the spirit. Do you feel and sense that part of you springing to life? Nourish that spirit. Cherish it. It is the life force inside you working for you, helping you get well again.

Decide. The decision comes first; the results follow. Today is the day. Now is the hour. This is the moment! Decide!

An Essential Thing You Can Do

Now, make the treatment decision. Appreciate the power of your commitment. Be optimistic. Decide! Inform your team of your choice.

#12

Give Only Informed Consent

All treatment decisions should be made—must be made—with the informed consent of the patient or patient's guardian. This means you need to know in detail, in terms you can clearly understand, all the risks entailed in any procedure involving surgery, anesthesia, radiation therapy, chemotherapy, or other medical encounters.

You'll be asked to sign a consent form. Do not sign a blank consent form. Make certain that the exact procedure is described and that you fully understand it. You have the right to set limits on these documents. You can cross out statements to which you do not consent. For example, I drew a line through the section of my consent form that asked my permission to videotape the operation for the removal of my lung.

You have the right to refuse treatment. An adult who is mentally competent can refuse treatment even if it may result in death. Nancy was a young woman who was pregnant. Even though she was advised to go ahead with treatment for lung cancer, she felt so strongly about the potential harm to her unborn child that she elected to postpone treatment until after her delivery. She exercised her right to refuse consent.

Your medical team is obligated to inform you fully of any procedure to which you are being asked to give consent. This means explaining to you the procedure's purpose, risks, other alternatives, and the risk involved in not having the procedure. Don't be intimidated by the medical lingo. Make certain you receive this information in language you understand.

More important, make certain you ask detailed questions prior to giving any consent. Please do not tolerate an attitude from anyone on your medical team that your concerns are unwelcome. And please be certain to include on your list of questions "Why is this absolutely necessary?"

An Essential Thing You Can Do

Ask your physician to describe clearly the risks involved in your tests and treatment. Compare the risks to the expected benefits. Only then can you give truly informed consent.

The Third Step on the Incredible Journey:
Manage Your Treatment

Breast cancer treatment can be a complex endeavor. There are many aspects to understand and coordinate. Ultimately, you are the one who needs to be in charge. This includes not only appointments and tests but also, most important, your self-care.

From making the most of your appointments to monitoring your progress to taking time for yourself, you—not the medical team—are the one who makes the real difference. Let's explore some simple and powerful ideas that will make treatment management easier.

#13

Believe in Your Treatment

Excited belief is one of the great intangibles in a successful breast cancer treatment program. It is a natural extension of your conviction about your treatment decisions. And it is your personal responsibility to believe in, and even be excited about, your treatment program.

Rachael and May both attended one of our seminars in Atlanta. Rachael is a Georgia homemaker who started a course of radiation following surgery for breast cancer. Her attitude toward treatment was "I guess it's something I have to do."

May received virtually the same diagnosis about a month after Rachael. May also had surgery and a follow-up course of chemotherapy. But her attitude was totally different from Rachael's: "I saw those chemicals as a great healing agent, something coming into my body to make me well. I welcomed my chemotherapy with open arms!"

Today May is free of cancer. Rachael continues to struggle.

Breast cancer survivors develop a confidence and an excited belief in their treatment programs that other patients do not possess. I am convinced that a correlation exists between the belief in one's treatment and the treatment's effectiveness. My observations of the importance of belief in cancer treatment lead me to respect the awesome power of the mind and the human spirit in the cancer journey.

Celeste is a California wife, mother, and now retired elementary school teacher. After three years of remission, she had a recurrence of breast cancer including liver and bone metastasis. Her doctors gave her less than a year to live. "I knew I was at the crossroads," said Celeste. "And when I learned that survivors held an excited belief about their treatment, I decided I needed to do the same."

You can observe excited and expectant belief in survivor after survivor. I fully realize my observations are only anecdotal evidence.

But I am convinced this hypothesis is correct. Excited belief. Cancer survival is a matter of involving both head and heart. I have seen beliefs and attitudes like May's and Celeste's make the difference in hundreds of cases. The correlation between belief in treatment and effectiveness of that treatment is very high.

A correlation exists between the belief in one's treatment and the treatment's effectiveness. My observations of the importance of belief in cancer treatment lead me to respect the awesome power of the mind and the human spirit in the cancer journey.

Someday, the scientific and medical communities will fully document the biological reality of this kind of optimism. In the meantime, please do not enter the debate. Instead, learn from the survivors and develop an excited belief about your treatment.

An Essential Thing You Can Do

Embrace your treatment program. See it as a friend. Believe it is there to help you. Excited belief is what you seek.

#14

Overcome Fatigue and Nausea

Extreme fatigue is reported by nearly 90 percent of breast cancer patients. It is present both during and after treatment. Worse, getting more sleep or rest often does not relieve the fatigue. In fact, cancer-related fatigue is one of the most profound and distressing long-term survival issues cancer patients face.

What can be done? Moderate exercise is the number one treatment for fatigue. In patient after patient, exercise was found to mitigate fatigue and lead to more restful and predictable sleep. You'll find more information on this important thing to do in "#27 Make Exercise Part of Your Recovery."

In addition, the popular dietary supplement ginseng relieves fatigue and boosts energy levels in many people with cancer. Researchers studied 282 people with breast, colon, and other types of cancer. They were randomly assigned to take 750 milligrams, 1,000 milligrams, or 2,000 milligrams of American ginseng or placebo daily for eight weeks. About 25 percent of those on the two highest doses reported their fatigue was "moderately or much better," compared with only 10 percent of those taking the lowest dose or a placebo. Also, energy levels were about twice as high in those taking the 1,000-milligram dose as those taking the placebo. People taking the two highest doses also reported generally feeling better, with improvements in mental, physical, and emotional well-being. And they said they were more satisfied with their treatment.

The researchers tested the Wisconsin species of American ginseng, which is different from Chinese ginseng and other forms of American ginseng sold in health food stores. The ginseng was powdered and given in capsule form. However, there is one concern: the question remains unanswered on interactions with some conventional medical treatments. I recommend you stop consumption of ginseng forty-eight hours prior to chemotherapy and wait seventy-two hours after administration before resuming.

One of the realities for about half of the cancer patients undergoing chemotherapy is nausea. While there are other side effects including hair loss, fatigue, and the decreased ability of the body to make red and white blood cells and platelets, nausea is typically the most uncomfortable. It may or may not include vomiting. Most patients can significantly improve this experience, but it takes some experimentation because everyone's body is different. Here are some suggestions:

- Ask your oncologist for antinausea medication. Compazine, Tigan, and Zofran are commonly prescribed. Try taking them thirty to sixty minutes before treatments.

- Use relaxation exercises, specifically the one featured in Appendix 5: "Meditation and Visualization."

- Eat smaller meals more often. Try six daily meals. For meal options, see "Breast Cancer Charities Sample Meal Plan: Four to Six 'Mini-Meals' a Day" in Appendix 1: "Sample Menus."

- Emphasize low-fat foods, especially fresh fruits.

- Limit liquids taken with meals. Drink no liquids in the hour before meals or the hour following meals. But be sure to take in enough liquids at other times. If you choose chemotherapy, your medical team will tell you to drink more liquids to ensure good urine flow and to minimize problems with your liver, kidneys, and bladder.

- Clear, cool liquids are recommended. Iced green tea, ginger ale, clear broths, Popsicles, or apple juice ice cubes are worth trying. Take all liquids slowly.

- Eat dry food such as crackers, toast, and popcorn—especially at the start of the day or at the first sign of nausea. Sorry, no butter on the popcorn.

- Eat salty foods. Avoid overly sweet foods.

- Do not lie down for two hours after eating. You can rest sitting up. Or if you simply must stretch out, prop a couple of pillows under your head to gain elevation.

- Sometimes loose clothing or fresh air will help control nausea.

- Ask your pharmacist about Travel-Eze or Sea-Band antinausea wristbands.

- Drink gingerroot tea steeped with peppermint.

- Goldenseal root may be helpful.

- Try hypnosis. Several small clinical trials have shown significant reductions in nausea and vomiting when hypnotherapy is introduced.

An Essential Thing You Can Do

Experiment. Clearly, there is no one-size-fits-all answer to fatigue and nausea. You'll need to try several of the suggested ideas. They have proven successful for many other cancer patients. One or more may be just the answer for which you have been searching.

#15

Make the Most of Your Appointments

Free and open communication between you and your healthcare team is one of the most important aspects of your breast cancer journey. You need to stay informed. You want feedback. But seldom is this information volunteered. You'll have to ask for it.

Wise patients bring a list of questions to virtually every medical appointment. If you have continuing or new symptoms, ask about them. If you are experiencing side effects, ask about them. Ask for further information about issues you have learned from your reading or from talking to other patients.

Speak with total honesty to your doctor and the entire healthcare team. They are not mind readers. Tell them your problems, and ask for their opinions. Bring a family member with you if you have trouble being assertive. He can be your wellness advocate. Many people are intimidated by their doctors. If you are one of these people, recognize it and act immediately to remove that needless hurdle. If you are having trouble understanding and absorbing medical information, bring an audio recorder. Then you'll be able to review explanations and instructions at your convenience.

Your ability to ask questions is one of your most significant points of power. When in doubt, write down your questions and then read them from your list.

In case this hasn't been emphasized enough by now, please understand that your ability to ask questions is one of your most significant points of power. When in doubt, write down your questions and then read them from your list.

One other insider's tip: If you truly want to make the most of your medical appointments, get in the habit of expressing your sincere gratitude to your medical team. One group of doctors at a large healthcare system in Pittsburgh lamented to me, "We try so earnestly to help a patient. I wish once in a while they would simply say thank you." I clearly remember giving an appreciative hug to my oncologist. From that day forward, I was treated like royalty in that office. Start showing your appreciation to these very important people in your life. Remember, they're people who respond to you just as you respond to them.

An Essential Thing You Can Do

In your Wellness and Recovery Journal, record both your questions and the answers you are given. Keep this information handy. Bring it to your appointments. If you rely on your memory, or record your questions on bits of paper scattered here and there, you'll never obtain timely and accurate information.

Write a thank-you note to at least one person on your medical team following your next visit.

#16

Monitor Your Progress

As you continue your treatment program, you'll be given tests to determine how well it's working. Ask about the tests prior to agreeing to them. Then insist that the doctor share the results.

It's uplifting to know that you are making progress. But even a report that is less encouraging can have a positive side. It should lead you and your doctor to consider other forms of treatment. Many exist. If all standard therapies have been exhausted, ask about investigative treatments. Or look more seriously at the complementary and alternative choices.

It is your responsibility to monitor your treatment program. Don't wait. Ask.

An Essential Thing You Can Do

Ask your doctor how and when he will check the progress of your treatment. Write this information in your Wellness and Recovery Journal. Then be certain tests occur as scheduled.

The Fourth Step on the Incredible Journey:
Heal Your Lifestyle

A Stanford University health newsletter estimated that lifestyle issues such as poor diet, lack of exercise, and unwise health habits accounted for 61 percent of premature deaths due to cancer. They estimated medical treatments themselves were listed as contributing to 10 percent of cancer deaths.

I believe these estimates are low, especially for breast cancer. As we previously discussed, the vitamin D evidence is overwhelming. It shows nearly eight of ten breast cancers can now be prevented. And if you already have breast cancer, we will shortly discuss how low-dose aspirin can help prevent recurrence. All this is good news. It means there is little question that you can influence both the onset of breast cancer and the progression of the disease.

Your lifestyle choices are critical in the breast cancer survival journey. These are under your control, a matter of intention, an issue of choice. Clearly, there is much you can do to help yourself get well and stay well. Let's examine how literally millions of women have helped in their own healing.

#17

Live Well

Make wellness your way of life. It's a stance one chooses in order to maximize one's health—physically, emotionally, and spiritually. Wellness recognizes the fact that everything one thinks, says, does, feels, and believes has an impact on your health and your life. Wellness can be chosen at any moment, in any circumstance. Wellness is possible even though you are diagnosed with breast cancer, even with metastatic disease.

Wellness can be chosen at any moment, in any circumstance. Wellness is possible even though you are diagnosed with breast cancer, even with metastatic disease.

Breast cancer survivorship is a combination of head and heart. Conquering demands that you reach beyond the physical issues of illness. Your mental, emotional, and spiritual health has a powerful effect on your well-being.

Isabelle was a thirty-eight-year-old attorney in Paris. A busy mother of three, she was now pregnant with her fourth child. The lump she felt in her left breast seemed to be consistent with her previous pregnancies. Her pediatrician felt otherwise. She ordered a biopsy, and the results confirmed breast cancer.

"I went through the treatments exactly as recommended," said Isabelle. "But I knew the real problem. I wasn't taking care of myself." With all the demands of work and family, there was no time for self-care.

Like so many survivors, Isabelle considered cancer her wake-up call. "I clearly needed to change."

Similar sentiments are expressed by thousands of survivors. They see illness as a message to make life changes. Isabelle's first move was to change her work schedule. She determined she would work only four days a week, leaving Wednesdays free. She arranged for at-home childcare rather than making a mad rush to the nursery school each morning. And on those days when she did work, Isabelle began to take a longer lunch hour so that she could go home to be with her children. "Changing my work and life balance was the reason I began to heal," she reflected. "Breast cancer put me on notice that I needed to live my life differently."

Living well, intentional choice, <u>exercising the decision to take personal responsibility for one's</u> total well-being—this is common talk among breast cancer survivors. It's whole-person wellness, a triumphant way of living. I want this so much for you.

Although wellness may be obscured by illness, it is a matter of personal choice whether wellness will be destroyed by illness. I am encouraging you to discover high-level wellness in the very midst of life-threatening illness. Wellness is not about the condition of being cured. It is about our awareness that every moment is a gift that we can savor.

Never again will your well-being be a static state measured simply by the lack of disease. Instead, wellness becomes your new way of living.

The decision to live well is significant and profound. Never again will your well-being be a static state measured simply by the lack of disease. Instead, wellness becomes your new way of living.

An Essential Thing You Can Do

Begin the wellness quest. Open your mind and spirit to whole-person wellness. In your Wellness and Recovery Journal, record one step you can take today to improve your greater well-being, such as "I am going to be happy—anyway!" Now please act on that idea. Do what is clearly doable today, this hour. <u>Decide to live your life at a new and higher</u> level of wellness no matter what.

#18

Operate Under New Assumptions

Compare the assumptions behind conventional healthcare with those behind whole-person wellness:

Assumptions behind Conventional Healthcare

1. The patient is reliant upon the medical community.
2. The professional is the authority.
3. Symptoms are treated, not investigated.
4. Treatment is specialized and concerned with the body's subsystems.
5. Breast cancer is a specific functional breakdown.
6. Primary repairs are made with surgery or drugs.
7. Pain and illness are purely negative.
8. Mind and emotions are a secondary factor in health.
9. Body and mind are separate. Spirit has no health impact.
10. Disease prevention is largely environmental: not smoking and paying careful attention to diet, exercise, and rest.

Assumptions behind Whole-Person Wellness

1. The patient has, or should develop, independence.
2. The professional is a healing partner.
3. The underlying causes are sought, and the symptoms are treated.
4. Treatment is unified and concerned with a person's whole life.
5. The body is as an ever-changing system.
6. Intervention is minimal and appropriate. Noninvasive therapies are used when possible.
7. Pain and illness are messages to value and act upon.

8. Mind and emotions are major factors in health.

9. Body, mind, and spirit form one unit and always affect each other.

10. *Wellness* means prevention plus wholeness: harmony in relationships, work, goals; a balance of body, mind, and spirit.

There is an exceedingly important principle behind these assumptions. Your medical team will be helpful in addressing just one part of your breast cancer journey, the physical disease portion. Wellness encompasses far more. Whole-person well-being is our goal, and the responsibility for achieving it falls to each of us.

An Essential Thing You Can Do

Review the above assumptions. Circle those you believe to be true. Are you a traditionalist? Do you identify with the spirit of whole-person wellness? What does this analysis tell you to do differently? Which assumptions serve you best? Breast cancer treatment is a lot more than medicine. Please view the breast cancer experience through the lens of the "whole you."

#19

Schedule Your Wellness

All important tasks demand a schedule. And there is no more important work in your life right now than the work of getting well again.

The trouble is, most people keep putting off the work of wellness, thinking they will get to it later. And guess what? They seldom, if ever, get around to it. Or if they do, it's only after everything else that is "important" has been accomplished.

Develop the attitude that there is nothing more important in your life right now than your work of wellness.

Develop the attitude that there is nothing more important in your life right now than your work of wellness. For the time being, your wellness efforts need to take priority over family, work, community or religious activities, and social obligations. Getting well is your new top priority. I gently encourage you to incorporate the disciplines of wellness into your daily life.

You may have your own techniques, but I actually blocked out my day on an appointment calendar. Here's what that schedule looked like while I was in the middle of recovery:

6:00 a.m.	Wake up
6:15 a.m.	Exercise
6:45 a.m.	Meditate
7:00 a.m.	Shower, eat, and commute
9:00 a.m.	Work
Noon	Lunch and meditate
1:00 p.m.	Work
4:30 p.m.	Commute
5:30 p.m.	Meditate
6:00 p.m.	Dinner

7:00 p.m.   Family time

9:00 p.m.   Read and meditate

10:00 p.m.   Sleep

Doctor appointments were worked in as needed. During commutes, I virtually always listened to wellness CDs. Weekends found me devoting even more time to study and meditation.

I encourage you to do something similar. Make a schedule that works for you, a guideline for your wellness program. The good news is that you can implement this schedule in a way that is gentle and less demanding of outside activities. You need not be a slave to your schedule. It should be a pattern of life that allows you more time for self-care. I encourage you now to take control of your days and make the work of wellness your top priority.

An Essential Thing You Can Do

Start a new page in your Wellness and Recovery Journal. Plan a schedule for your week. Minimize obligations that cause undue stress. Give ample core time to the wellness disciplines discussed in this book.

. . . .

Take a Break

After completing your schedule, I suggest you take a break from your wellness work. Start the next section tomorrow or after you have rested. In the meantime, give careful consideration to how you spend your time. Please understand that I am asking you to make wellness a way of life. For most people, this means a major lifestyle shift. Look within. Consider the evidence and the implications of these suggestions. Begin now to modify your schedule to meet your new wellness priorities.

#20

Eliminate Active and
Passive Smoking

Please don't smoke. And don't be near people while they are smoking.

Do you know that this recommendation is different from the position of the American Cancer Society, the Canadian Cancer Society, and Cancer Research UK? These very large and cash-rich not-for-profit organizations claim there is insufficient evidence of smoking's causal link to breast cancer. Incredible. It's a classic case of the blind limits of the purely scientific model.

The fact is, there is evidence from new studies suggesting that smoking increases the risk of breast cancer. In addition, there is further scientific evidence that young women and girls face special risks from exposure to smoke. Thankfully, the *New York Times* reported that smoking, and even secondhand smoke exposure during adolescence, increases the risk of breast cancer occurring later in life.

Women who start smoking when they are young increase their risk of breast cancer by 20 percent, and many years of heavy smoking could increase the risk by up to 30 percent. In 2009, a panel of U.S. and Canadian researchers reviewed more recent studies. The panelists found "strong support" that smoking, and even secondhand smoke, increased the risk of premenopausal breast cancer.

Of course, this says nothing of the greater risk of developing lung cancer.

It completely mystifies me how some breast cancer patients can continue to use tobacco. We worked with a breast cancer patient from Toronto. When I discovered she was a pack-a-day smoker, I suggested she make it a priority to quit. Her response was "I enjoy smoking. Besides, I don't have lung cancer."

If I could communicate this any more strongly, I would. Stop smoking! If you are a user, please stop any and all tobacco use immediately. There is no excuse, even nicotine addiction, that is sufficient to continue this harmful habit. Come to the vivid realization that smoking is putting cancer-causing chemicals into your body.

A family practitioner recently shared with me that he was not going to tell his patients to stop smoking. I was stunned and said, "What?!" "Some of them enjoy a cigarette," he said. "And besides, I don't want to offend them." My response was that smokers know they should quit, most want to quit, and, far from being offended, they want their doctor to help them quit.

The question is not whether you can quit. The question is whether you will quit. I know this firsthand. I started smoking when I was in my teens. There is no doubt that smoking directly contributed to my lung cancer just over twenty years later. In those twenty years, I seriously tried to quit five or six times. Willpower alone didn't get the job done. A change in my thinking did.

It started with changing my self-perception. I first went from perceiving myself as a smoker to seeing myself as a person who mistakenly chose the behavior of smoking. Seeing smoking as a behavior helped me detach emotionally and psychologically from the cigarettes. I was then able to perceive myself as a nonsmoker. If you are a smoker, a similar change in self-image can work for you, too. From this moment forward, see yourself as a nonsmoker.

It started with changing my self-perception. I first went from perceiving myself as a smoker to seeing myself as a person who mistakenly chose the behavior of smoking.

In addition to never smoking again, I ask you to eliminate your exposure to passive smoking. A Finnish study revealed up to a one-third drop in circulating levels of vitamin C and other antioxidants after just thirty minutes of exposure to secondhand smoke.

It has never been more important for you to maximize your health. Tobacco use and exposure to secondhand smoke have no place in your quest for living well.

An Essential Thing You Can Do

Stop all tobacco use immediately. Envision yourself as completely tobacco free. Wean yourself with a nicotine patch if you must. But get that self-image of being a nonsmoker deep into your soul. And stay away from tobacco users while they are smoking.

#21
Adopt This Nutritional Strategy

During a counseling session with Cara, a breast cancer patient in her midfifties, her interest quickly turned to nutrition. "Can you describe your diet?" I asked. Cara's reply was, "My doctor says I can eat anything I like. And he doesn't want me to lose weight."

That may have been medical advice, but it was not an informed medical opinion. The days of "eat anything you want" are long gone. In fact, that philosophy may have contributed to the onset of Cara's cancer. It certainly detracts from maximizing Cara's health and well-being.

The field of nutritional science is notorious for its lack of definitive answers. As nutritionists will be only too glad to tell you, more research must be done. But there is a great deal we do know about nutrition and its links to our health. In more than twenty-five years of work in this field, I have learned two important principles, things you need to know about the link between diet and cancer, which are not in contention among the nutritional gurus:

Fact 1: The Western diet invariably results in the Western diseases.

The Western diet is typically defined as a diet that is composed of lots of processed foods and meats and contains significant amounts of added sugars, fats, salts, and preservatives, as well as a lot of refined grains. This diet minimizes and even leaves out fresh vegetables, fresh fruits, and whole grains.

The inevitable result of this Western diet is that the population suffers from high rates of obesity, diabetes, cardiovascular disease, and cancer. Credible research indicates nearly all the obesity and type 2 diabetes cases, more than 80 percent of the cardiovascular diseases, and at least half of cancers in the United States are linked to this diet. Sound familiar?

Fact 2: People who eat more natural diets suffer far less from the Western diseases.

While there is no single diet that can be prescribed for disease prevention and recovery, this much is clear: those who eat minimal amounts of trans fats, maintain a high ratio of polyunsaturated to saturated fats, enjoy six or more servings of fresh vegetables and fruits per day, consume high amounts of whole grains, and have two or three servings of fish per week have lower rates of the Western diseases.

The hopeful fact is that people who switch from the Western diet to the natural diet see significant improvements in health. In the process, they help prevent the onset of the typical Western diseases.

Previously, we briefly discussed this nutritional strategy. Let's review. Here are the most common nutritional shifts employed by hundreds-of-thousands of cancer survivors:

- Eating whole foods
- Minimizing fat, salt, and sugar
- Emphasizing fresh vegetables, fresh fruits, and whole grains

The single most important dietary shift is consuming foods that are less processed. If it is boxed or bottled or canned or packaged, the food comes under immediate scrutiny. Prepared foods, even when enriched, tend to deliver calories with less nutrition than their fresh counterparts. This means cancer survivors spend most of their grocery shopping time in the produce section of their local market.

Whole Foods

Whole foods include fresh vegetables, fresh fruits, whole grains, whole grain pastas, brown rice, raw nuts, sprouted breads, and the like. See the Breast Cancer Charities Shopping List that follows in Appendix 4.

Low Fat, Salt, and Sugar

Good fats like unsaturated fats are often classified into two groups: the omega-3s and the omega-6s. They come from extra-virgin olive oil, sesame oil, seeds—especially flaxseed—and fatty fish.

Low salt means the right salt—sea salt or the use of liquid aminos.

Low sugar means no added sugar. Sugar should come exclusively from whole food sources, and then only in moderation.

The issue of sugar requires a deeper understanding. I want to impress upon you the importance of avoiding refined sugar. The scientists call sugar an "obligate glucose metabolizer." Loosely translated, that means a "feeder." There exists significant evidence-based research pointing to sugar as doing two things that stand in the way of cancer recovery: The first is that sugar suppresses immune function. Second, it feeds the cancer cells.

> *Understand this next key point: one of insulin's multiple functions is to promote cell growth—be that normal healthy cells or malignant cells.*

Diets high in sugar, and foods that turn into sugar when digested, cause blood sugar levels to rise. Once this spike is triggered, the body releases a hormone called insulin in an effort to bring the blood sugar levels back to normal. Understand this next key point: one of insulin's multiple functions is to promote cell growth—be that normal healthy cells or malignant cells. Therefore, the more insulin circulating in the body, the more opportunity for cancer cells to be fed and in turn to grow and divide.

This leads to a handy dietary guideline: "Whites out. Colors in."

"Whites out" mean to eliminate the following:

white sugar

white potatoes

white rice

white bread

white pasta

All these are simple carbohydrates that turn directly into sugar once ingested. The days of a couple of teaspoons of sugar in your coffee or sprinkled on your bowl of boxed cereal are over. Please, if you wish to prevent and survive breast cancer, take the whites out!

"Colors in" means to add fresh vegetables of many colors, including:

broccoli

kale

parsley

cabbage

romaine and leaf lettuce

spinach

peppers

cauliflower

beets

leeks

sweet potatoes

and fresh fruits of many colors, including:

tomatoes (they are a fruit)

apples

lemons

grapes

blueberries

Whites out. Colors in. It's a simple and very achievable dietary strategy.

We recommend consuming fruits in lesser quantities than vegetables. The sugar content in fruit is comparatively high.

Whites out. Colors in. It's a simple and very achievable dietary strategy. There has never been a more important time in your life to eat well. Eating whole foods, minimizing fat, salt, and sugar, and emphasizing fresh fruits and vegetables and whole grains—it's your new nutritional program.

An Essential Thing You Can Do

This is just a decision. So decide. Your decision to eat healthfully, better than ever before in your entire life, will help ensure your maximum opportunity to survive and thrive following a breast cancer diagnosis.

#22

Purchase Real Food

The purpose of this section is to communicate in a clear, practical, and useful manner the best food choices. The best way I know how to do this is by giving you specific recommendations that are good as well as not so good. All nutritional education is useless unless and until it is applied. And this clear choice list a very good way to apply this knowledge.

The foods on this Green Light List pass the test. The passing grade is based on an analysis of the food's nutrient density. Nutrient density takes into account vitamins, minerals, protein, fiber, healthy fats content, plus glycemic index and calories.

Green Light List

Vegetables	Fruits
broccoli	berries
cabbage	oranges
peppers	red grapefruit
carrots	apples
leaf lettuce	cherries
cauliflower	apricots
onions	cantaloupe
beets	kiwi
asparagus	pears
squash	red grapes
pumpkin	watermelon
	tomatoes

Fish and Meat	Whole Grains and Breads
cod	oats
flounder	oatmeal
tilapia	barley
salmon (wild)	brown rice
tuna	flaxseed
trout	buckwheat
mahi-mahi	spelt wheat
sardines	millet
haddock	amaranth
skinless chicken breast	pita bread
turkey breast	wheat germ

Legumes	Other
black beans	garlic
garbanzo beans	ginger
kidney beans	cinnamon
navy beans	cayenne
pinto beans	stevia
lentils	green tea
split peas	curry

Nonfat Dairy	Oils
yogurt	extra-virgin olive oil
cottage cheese	sesame oil
almond milk	nonfat vegetable spray

On the opposite end of the spectrum, there are several foods that clearly do not receive a passing grade. They deliver calories with few nutrients. This is the Red Light List. If you are in active treatment for breast cancer, please do not put these foods in your mouth.

sugar	liquor
aspartame	beer
syrups	wine
hydrogenated fats	soft drinks, regular and diet
lard	honey
margarine	ice cream
salami	cookies
hot dogs	doughnuts
bologna	cake
sausage	boxed cereal
bacon	molasses
smoked ham	mayonnaise
pizza	

This does not mean you can never have another piece of pizza in your life. It does mean that this is the time in your life to eat real food, meaning whole foods that are nutrient dense and low in fat, salt, and sugar, and that emphasize fresh vegetables, fresh fruits, and whole grains.

The good news is that there is an endless combination of menu items based on these nutrient-dense foods. So be creative. Experiment with your menu. You will be contributing to your health and well-being in a major way.

An Essential Thing You Can Do

There has never been a more important time in your life to eat well. If you are in the middle of cancer treatment, hold yourself accountable for eating from the approved Green Light shopping list. See Appendix 4: "The Real Food Shopping List" in the Food as Medicine appendixes for the Green Light food choices in shopping-list form.

#23

Hydrate

Drink lots of pure water. It's a simple and effective way to vastly increase your opportunity for breast cancer prevention, survival, and recovery. Drink the equivalent of eight cups of water each and every day! Not coffee. Not soda. Not juice. Water.

It is an almost universal truth—women with breast cancer are dehydrated. Lack of water inhibits immune function, the most potent defense you have against cancer. The environment in which your cells live is not blood; it is fluid. The lymph system, a key component of your immune system, is a fluid system requiring adequate water to function at its highest capacity.

Through natural elimination, perspiration, and even breathing, your body loses fluids. Fluid must be continually replaced in appropriate quantities for you to be optimally well.

The environment in which your cells live is not blood; it is fluid.

In addition, you need more water if

- You are exercising
- The weather is hot
- You perspire a lot—including the sweats from chemotherapy
- You have a fever
- You have diarrhea or are vomiting

I prefer water with no chlorine or fluorides. This is difficult to obtain from most municipal water systems. About two of three municipal water supplies in America still contain both chlorine and fluoride, chemicals long known to cause cancer. Even bottled water, especially if contained in plastic, is not a sure answer. Some research indicates that sunlight starts a chemical reaction in the plastic bottle that can result in carcinogens in the water.

How can you obtain pure water? I recommend using a water purification system in your home or purchasing certified chemical-free, spring-fed bottled water in glass containers.

An Essential Thing You Can Do
Drink eight cups of pure water each day.

#24

Know Why You Eat

Long-term dietary changes require more than shifts in our menus. Our food preferences are a factor of culture and habit. Our enjoyment of food is so much a part of our lives that any permanent change is best supported by not only choosing *what we eat* but also understanding *why we eat*.

I like to think I am not alone in this behavior. On countless occasions, I have allowed my frame of mind, rather than my body, to determine my food choices. Comfort foods to satisfy our emotions, to soothe our anger, frustration, worry, boredom, or guilt, are most often the culprit. Have you noticed how relief from stress is easily accomplished by eating? I have. And when this happens, we have linked food to emotional fulfillment. This is dangerous territory. You and I would be better served if we cultivated a heightened awareness of why we eat.

Eating with awareness is easily accomplished with the help of these proven practices:

- Don't keep any high-fat snack foods around the house where they will be a serious temptation.

- Make a rule of not eating in front of the television, where you don't pay attention to what or how much you eat.

- Don't eat so quickly that you can't enjoy your food. It takes about twenty minutes for our brains to realize that our stomachs are full. Slow down. Take a break midmeal.

- Reward appropriate eating behavior, but don't use comfort foods as the reward. If you've had a good week or have reached a health goal, treat yourself to a movie, a concert, or a new outfit. Don't punish imperfection, just don't reward yourself. Try again next week.

- Make each meal a pleasant experience. Stop eating on the run or while standing at the kitchen counter. Take time to put out a place setting. Offer a short affirmation or prayer of gratitude for each meal. You'll then be nurturing yourself emotionally and spiritually as well as physically.

An Essential Thing You Can Do

Join me. Let's become experts at distinguishing between a food craving, which is a psychological need, and hunger, which is the body's need for nourishment. Check your urge to eat the next time you see a food advertisement. A craving diminishes when we take on another activity. Go for a walk. Call a friend. Read a book. Then evaluate. Were you feeling a craving or hunger? Honor your hunger, not your craving. Eat with awareness!

#25

Determine Your Nutritional Supplement Program

Please, please, please, if you have breast cancer, implement the following nutritional supplement strategy today.

Each day, consume 5,000 IU of vitamin D_3 and 1,000 mg of calcium citrate. Arrange for a monthly blood test. Add more vitamin D until you reach and maintain what is called the 25(OH)D at a level of 55–60 ng/mL. If you are one of the very few women who are hypercalcemic, eliminate the calcium supplementation.

If you do not have breast cancer, you'll want to maximize prevention. Therefore, consume 2,000 IU of vitamin D_3 each day. Test blood levels annually to maintain a vitamin D level of 30–40 ng/mL.

If you do not have breast cancer, you'll want to maximize prevention. Therefore, consume 2,000 IU of vitamin D_3 each day.

This simple program is of critical importance to your health and recovery from breast cancer. As we have already explored, there is excellent science to back this recommendation.

Let's understand the context of nutritional supplements. All essential nutrients are important for rebuilding and maintaining health. But obtaining those through diet alone is very difficult. Today we have compelling research that shows the following to be particularly beneficial to people with cancer.

Antioxidants

Vitamins C and E and mixed carotenoids, a precursor of vitamin A, work best in combination. They are especially beneficial in combating the effects of free radical damage to DNA. Selenium is an essential mineral that is an important part of antioxidant activity. Coenzyme Q_{10} is an antioxidant compound made naturally by the body and used by cells to produce controlled cell growth and mainte-nance. However, when the body's immune function is compromised, the body's natural ability to produce CoQ_{10} is often impaired.

Carotenoids

Carotenoids are a class of natural pigments found principally in plants, algae, and certain bacteria. They have antioxidant activity, and some, such as beta-carotene, are converted to vitamin A by the body. Lycopene is also a particularly beneficial carotenoid for the prevention of and natural treatment for cancer. Fresh organic toma-toes are a rich source of lycopene. In order to maximize absorption, tomatoes are best eaten lightly cooked, then pureed and topped with a splash of extra-virgin olive oil.

Flavonoids

Like carotenoids, flavonoids are one of the groups of plant nutrients with powerful antioxidant characteristics as well as other cancer-fighting properties.

Omega-3 Fatty Acids

Three omega-3 fatty acids—ALA (alpha-linolenic acid), DHA (docosahexaenoic acid), and EPA (eicosapentaenoic acid)—are essential to good health. For cancer patients, the fats are particularly important because they support immune function and hormone bal-ance. The best source of the omega-3s is oily fish, including wild salmon, tuna, mackerel, and sardines. For people unable or choosing not to eat fish, flaxseed can be a good source of fatty acid. However, flaxseed oil does not contain DHA or EPA. Some brands now add DHA from a plant source.

Probiotics

This is a supplement of beneficial bacteria that promotes gastroin-testinal balance. One example is lactobacillus acidophilus. Many cancer treatments are notorious for causing nausea and diarrhea.

Most patients can find relief by rebalancing the intestinal tract with probiotics to maintain digestive health.

Most breast cancer survivors believe in and use vitamin and mineral supplements. Despite their bad reputation in medical circles, vitamin and mineral supplements can and should be effectively used, not avoided, even during breast cancer treatment.

Along with a dietary strategy that includes whole foods, fresh vegetables, and fresh fruits and minimizes fat, salt, and sugar, vitamin and mineral supplements form the basis for the Breast Cancer Charities "Eat Well" approach to nutrition. The program is designed to guide and support people in ways to maximize strengthening the body and promoting an optimally functioning immune system.

Exhaustive and credible research shows that the right levels of nutrients are both protective against developing many cancers and supportive of health and healing following a diagnosis.

Ideally, we should receive all our nutrients from our food. But even with the best diet, this is often not possible. Intensive farming practices have led to a demonstrated decline in the nutritional value of certain foods. And even upon implementing the real food diet that we previously discussed, it still may not be possible to receive all the nutrients you need in the right amounts all the time.

Ideally, we should receive all our nutrients from our food. But even with the best diet, this is often not possible.

In addition, significant evidence reveals the negative health impact of the wide range of chemicals we are exposed to in everyday life, even in our fresh and prepared foods. This calls for an even greater need for nutrients to help with detoxification and protection.

Below, you will find specific guidelines that contain information about vitamins, minerals, and other nutritional supplements, along with recommended dosages, that are thought to be specifically supportive for people who have had a cancer diagnosis. Cancer Recovery Group, the parent organization of Breast Cancer Charities of America, developed this program based on research and information from around the world. The goal is to provide a full range of essential nutrients with an emphasis on obtaining maximum absorption and bioavailability.

For those women who wish to promote health and healing, three guidelines on nutritional supplements stand out:

- For breast cancer prevention and treatment, vitamin D and calcium supplementation is the minimal starting point. In my opinion, every woman should be on these supplements.

- Next in importance are the antioxidants that prevent damage caused by excess free radicals in your body, the highly reactive chemicals that can damage your DNA or increase the expression of genetic predispositions in cells.

- Unless otherwise stated on the label, supplements are best taken with food. This helps maximize absorption.

I am frequently asked why the vitamin and mineral doses the Cancer Recovery Group suggests are higher than the government's recommendations, called dietary reference intakes (DRI). The DRI is often set at the level that prevents a deficiency disease, scurvy for example. But this does not necessarily mean that same level will be adequate for supporting maximum health, cancer prevention, or rebuilding a cancer patient's immune system. Cancer Recovery's guidelines meet standards above disease deficiency and therefore must be higher than the DRI guidance.

Taking supplements during cancer treatment is a subject of intense debate within the cancer community. Cancer Recovery Group carefully monitors research on this subject, constantly updating our recommendations. Following consultation with your oncologist, we recommend the following:

If you are on a chemotherapy regimen:

- Suspend your supplement program two days (forty-eight hours) prior to treatment

- Recommence your supplement program three days (seventy-two hours) following treatment

- If you are on a continuous infusion treatment protocol, do not take supplements during active treatment

If you are on a radiation therapy or hormonal therapy regimen, continue to take supplements during treatment.

I recommend that all people with a personal history of cancer take supplements for the balance of their life. Evidence is clear that proper nutrient levels translate to maximizing health and maintaining healing. In addition, we recommend that people taking supplements over their lifetime have regular appointments with a nutritional therapist and regularly visit *www.thebreastcancercharities.org* for the most up-to-date nutritional guidelines.

I am also frequently asked, "What brand name of supplements is best?" I do not have a good answer. I simply recommend you choose the highest-quality supplements available. The best supplements will contain fewer nonactive ingredients such as preservatives and binding agents. Higher-quality supplements are also less likely to contain artificial sweeteners and coloring. While this level of supplement tends to be more expensive, I believe the incremental expense to be proportional to the supplement's value.

Every three months, Cancer Recovery Group monitors no less than sixteen different sources in twelve countries to review research findings on nutritional supplement guidelines.

Some cancer patients have difficulty swallowing tablets. In fact, "pill burden" is experienced by approximately 15 percent of cancer patients. Simple techniques resolve nearly all these difficulties. Large tablets can be crushed. Capsules can be pierced, although lycopene products may stain the teeth. Many vitamins and minerals can be obtained in liquid and powder form. If your concern is complete absorption of the nutrients, choose sublingual products, which are designed to be absorbed under the tongue.

Finally, keep up to date on nutritional supplement guidelines. Every three months, Cancer Recovery Group monitors no less than

Cancer Recovery Group's Nutritional Supplement Guidelines

Nutrient	Details	Daily Dose	Comments
multivitamin and mineral	highest quality	as directed	try to avoid preservatives, binders, and sweeteners
vitamin B	in addition to multivitamin and mineral complex	50–100 mg	
vitamin C with flavonoids	nonacidic ascorbate forms or with food	2,000 mg/2 g	take amounts over 1 g in divided doses with meals
vitamin D$_3$	in addition to multivitamin and mineral complex	5,000 mg	see chapter 5
vitamin E* (natural form in mixed tocopherols)	as part of a multivitamin and mineral complex	400 IU	best taken with vitamin C and beta-carotene
mixed carotenoids	in addition to multivitamin and mineral complex	25,000 IU	if you smoke, or have smoked in the past ten years, do not take more than 1,000 IU daily
calcium citrate		1,000 mg	do not take calcium if you're hypercalcemic
lycopene	maximum of 7 g	10–15 mg	do not take carrot juice at the same time

Nutrient	Details	Daily Dose	Comments
omega-3 fatty acids	fish oils	EPA + DHA 500 mg or more	whole fish oil; no cod oil, which may contain mercury
	or flaxseed oil with DHA	1,000 mg	alternative for those who don't eat or are allergic to fish
selenium	in addition to multivitamin and mineral complex	200 mcg	
zinc	in addition to multivitamin and mineral complex	20 mg	
coenzyme Q_{10}	protects heart during chemotherapy	100 mg	
probiotics	for digestive disorder (nausea, diarrhea)	1 or 2 capsules, as directed	minimum 1 billion organisms; keep refrigerated
milk thistle	for liver health during treatment	200 mg twice daily	

* Special note on vitamin E: If you have high blood pressure, are taking warfarin, aspirin, or any other antithrombotic drug, are on a chemotherapy regimen, or have a low platelet count, consult your doctor before taking more than 200 IU daily. This vitamin has a mild anticoagulant effect.)

sixteen different sources in twelve countries to review research findings on this important subject. We then review our recommendations and update them when evidence supports such changes.

An Essential Thing You Can Do

Do your homework. Contact a professional nutritionist. Determine what specific experience she has in therapeutic nutritional supplementation for cancer. Compare the nutritionist's recommendations with Cancer Recovery Group's recommendations as well as your own research. Be skeptical of unsubstantiated claims. Then, make your own decisions regarding nutritional supplements.

Do your homework. Contact a professional nutritionist.

Notice: Greg Anderson and Cancer Recovery Foundation make every effort to use up-to-date and reliable sources. However, we cannot accept liability for errors in the sources that we use. Also, we cannot guarantee to provide all the information that may be available concerning your individual health circumstances. All responsibility for interpretation of and action upon the information provided is yours. This information is offered on the understanding that if you intend to support your cancer treatment with complementary or alternative approaches, you will consult with your medical team to be certain they have a complete understanding of your choices.

#26

Take One Low-Dose Aspirin
Each Day

Beyond vitamin D, evidence points to something as simple as aspirin has a role in preventing breast cancer recurrence.

"Has it spread? Am I going to die?" Those are the frightening questions that invariably run through the minds of women who have been told that they have breast cancer. After they courageously take on surgery, long and arduous chemotherapy, and radiation treatments, the last group they want to join is the forty thousand women whose breast cancer will take a deadly turn and relapse, often relentlessly spreading throughout their body.

A report from the Nurses' Health Study offers women who have had breast cancer some vital and actionable information. Taking a single aspirin tablet—a baby aspirin—every day can be lifesaving. As reported in *U.S. News & World Report*, "were these aspirin tablets a hot new biotech drug, we would be popping champagne right now." Long-term, low-dose aspirin initiated a year or more after the cancer diagnosis as an add-on to treatment, not as a substitute for it, seems to help manage the tumor cells silently left behind.

> *Taking a single aspirin tablet— a baby aspirin— every day can be lifesaving.*

The study followed 4,164 breast cancer survivors over a period from 1976 to 2006, assessing in detail their use of aspirin. The women studied initially presented with tumors ranging from small, early-invasive cancers confined to the breast to more advanced ones that had spread into surrounding lymph nodes. Over more than three decades of follow-up, 400 of these women had a cancer recurrence with distant tumor spread, which had killed 341 of them by the time the study ended.

The power to spread is the power to kill, and what aspirin seems to be doing is interfering with that process. It was by coincidence, not by design, that almost half of the women in the study were diligently taking aspirin. The surprise finding: those who made aspirin a regular habit, consuming low doses two to five times a week, mostly to help their hearts, were 71 percent less likely to have a recurrence of their breast cancer compared to those who were taking little or no aspirin.

An Essential Thing You Can Do

If you wish to help prevent your breast cancer from spreading, take one baby aspirin each day. The typical active ingredient of children's aspirin is 81 mg per tablet.

#27

Make Exercise Part of Your Recovery Program

Being physically active significantly boosts the odds that you will survive the disease. Breast Cancer Charities of America has held this position from inception. Now we have several studies that show that exercise improves the prospects of beating any malignancy.

As we earlier discussed, a large, well-respected study of U.S. nurses found that breast cancer patients who walk or do other kinds of moderate exercise for three to five hours a week are about 50 percent less likely to die from the disease than sedentary women are.

Cancer survivors are markedly diverse in their exercise goals. Very few set out to run a marathon or become Olympic athletes. Instead, the most common exercise goal among cancer survivors is to experience an increase in energy.

Here's my exercise story. You may find this helpful in designing your own program.

The second day after surgery, while still in the hospital's intensive care unit, I began my exercise program. I first wrote a note to the nurse saying that I wanted to get off the ungodly ventilator that was doing my breathing. And within a couple of hours, I asked to be taken off the catheter, saying, "I can make it to the bathroom on my own." Both requests were granted by my surgeon, the same one who later told me he thought I had about thirty days to live.

I then asked if I could go for a walk around ICU. So using what we called the Christmas tree with three IVs hanging on it, the nurse accompanied me on a short, slow stroll. The next day, I tried to walk down the hall alone. That was too much.

So I began with chair exercises, doing simple arm circles—the backstroke movement with my arms fully extended. I'd do ten sets clockwise and follow with ten sets in the reverse direction. Soon I felt that increase in energy—the deeper breathing, the increase in heart rate, and the better skin color.

It wasn't long before I began to feel stronger. It seemed exercise was working. So I added a few minutes of leg lifts. Soon I was strong enough to put walking back into my exercise routine. Initially, I walked for perhaps five minutes before feeling an increase in energy. But soon that time stretched to ten minutes.

Over the months, the exercise periods became longer. I bought an exercise book and added some stretches before the start of my walk. I ended the exercise session with some light calisthenics. I began to feel the combination of physical and emotional regeneration working together to enhance my well-being.

Today, I believe I have found the right balance. Hardly a day passes that I do not walk for at least forty minutes. I precede the walk with about three minutes of warm-up stretches and conclude the session with five minutes of push-ups and sit-ups.

You can develop a similar program. Mine did not happen overnight. I determined this to be my correct level over a period of two years. Several times, I have experimented with exercise beyond the normal forty-minute daily routine. I tried walking for an hour each day but found I was experiencing hip soreness. I tried weight lifting only to realize I didn't enjoy it.

Make exercise part of your breast cancer recovery program. No matter how long it has been since you have exercised, no matter how incapacitated or confined you are, there are exercises you can do. Exercise will help you get well and stay well.

Some people think more exercise is better. A gentleman recently wrote me to express his opinion that two hours of intense exercise each day is a requirement for cancer recovery. I don't recommend it. Between the threat of injury associated with extended exercise and the rigid, grinding routine that often results in burnout, I believe more harm than good can come from workouts that last two or three hours daily.

Instead, I recommend you find a type of exercise that you enjoy. Then practice that routine just until you feel an increased flexibility and a sense of elation. And the psychological benefits are even greater—joy, enthusiasm, and mental vitality. What a payoff!

Make exercise part of your breast cancer recovery program. No matter how long it has been since you have exercised, no matter how incapacitated or confined you are, there are exercises you can do. Exercise will help you get well and stay well.

An Essential Thing You Can Do

Exercise just until you feel an increase in energy. This is your only exercise goal. Do the same tomorrow. Keep extending the duration as you build strength and stamina. No more excuses! Take charge. Your body will respond to your get-well signals. I know for certain that you can do this! I believe in you!

#28

Sleep More

Fatigue. It's the most common complaint of all cancer patients. "I'm always so tired. My radiation treatments drain me," noted Olivia during her recovery from breast cancer. "I just want to sleep all the time. But with all my responsibilities, who has time to sleep?"

Fatigue is part of nearly every breast cancer patient's experience. Unfortunately, many patients interpret fatigue as an indication of their fast-approaching demise. This is not necessarily so.

Many patients interpret fatigue as an indication of their fast-approaching demise. This is not necessarily so.

During and just after treatment, you are a different person physically. Just consider what is happening to you. With surgery, a major wound has been inflicted on your body. Chemotherapy puts chemicals into your system that alter your unique biochemical makeup. Radiation causes genetic and cellular changes in your body. Repairs demand rest. No wonder breast cancer patients are tired.

Survivors rest. Give yourself permission to take a daily nap. Even a couple of naps in the first few months. The fact is, survivors rest. It is a major mistake to carry on at the same frantic pace to which you were accustomed when you were supposedly healthy. Feeling tired is normal for anyone with any illness. During treatment, you may feel tired for weeks until your body gets the opportunity to adjust and recover. So allow yourself rest.

Provided you are obtaining adequate food and participating in moderate exercise, fatigue is nothing to consume you with worry. It is not a sure sign of your demise. Take that morning nap. Add an afternoon nap if you require it. Or a short rest before dinner may be just what is needed. Eight or more hours of sleep each night is an absolute essential.

An Essential Thing You Can Do

Give yourself permission to get more sleep. Block out rest times on your wellness schedule. Allow your body the rest it needs to repair and heal.

#29

Find Positive Support

You need a group of supportive family and friends. Consider this evidence: breast cancer patients who regularly participate in support group meetings live longer than those who do not.

Ongoing research at Stanford University confirmed what cancer survivors have known for decades. In a study of patients with advanced breast cancer, those who attended a weekly two-hour support group session had a life expectancy twice that of the non-attenders. Further research at UCLA and King's College in London confirms the value of attending support groups. The message is clear: we truly need one another for survival.

The message is clear: we truly need one another for survival.

Distinguish between the two major types of support groups: clinical and psychosocial. The clinical groups communicate basic knowledge on a wide variety of medical issues. Topics might include types of breast cancer treatments, common side effects, physical therapy following breast surgery, or how to live with a lymphedema. The idea behind this type of support group is to educate and inform.

More critical to survival are the psychosocial support groups. These are the supportive/expressive therapeutic programs that focus on the emotional, psychological, and spiritual aspects of cancer. Look for groups that take a stance of hope without denying the reality of the illness. At meetings, you should expect to express your own fears and frustrations freely and allow others in the group to do the same. You'll learn from the responses of the group members who have overcome cancer, and you'll contribute to those who are just beginning the cancer recovery journey.

One warning: A potential problem with any type of support group is that instead of encouraging personal growth, many groups quickly turn into a pity party. While there is significant value in allowing people to talk out their problems, the discerning group needs a leader to judge when the talking is therapeutic and when it is rehearsing, and reinforcing, a problem. The cyber solace provided in online chat groups is no exception.

In the mid-1980s, when a group of us started Cancer Conquerors support groups, committing to support one another in our healing quests, we made a pact early on. Each meeting would include a lesson—somebody leading a discussion on a recovery principle—and a time for open discussion and support. The emphasis was to be on the application of lessons that would help contribute to creating health. It was the smartest move we ever made. We have experienced very few pity parties.

An Essential Thing You Can Do

Visit *www.thebreastcancercharities.org* and view the full schedule of telesupport groups. Participate in several. Judge for yourself which groups work best for you.

If you don't find what you are looking for, perhaps you need to consider starting a group in your home. Thousands of patients have done so, benefiting themselves and others in their community. Contact Breast Cancer Charities of America and request the free booklet *How to Organize and Lead a Cancer Support Group*.

The Fifth Step on the Incredible Journey: Heal with Your Mind

Do our personal beliefs, positive attitudes, and hopeful expectations make a contribution to cancer recovery? A great deal of credible scientific evidence says yes. In fact, the contribution may be greater than science has the ability to measure.

Fighting cancer is much, much more than simply excising a tumor, exposing a malignancy to radiation, or administering chemotherapy through an intravenous drip.

Think bigger. Imagine harnessing all your resources, including the mind-body connection. The basics are actually quite simple. Let's continue our work.

#30

Analyze Your Beliefs

By now, you have been on the incredible breast cancer journey for some time. It is my hope that you have made your decisions on the treatment programs that have your conviction. Further, that you have adopted the nutrition and exercise protocols that help create high-level health and wellness. Most important, I trust that you have come to understand that you have the central role in this journey.

We are at the point where many breast cancer patients end their journey. I have just worked with Lin-Sy, a breast cancer patient from China now living in Canada. She has decided her time with us has come to an end. Lin-Sy shared, "In my culture, we value tradition. My husband and children need me. I have had my treatment. Now I want to get back to normal." Despite my reservations, I remained silent and wished her well.

You don't want your life to get back to normal. Normal was the environment where breast cancer was germinated. You want change for the better. And this portion of the breast cancer journey is where that profound transformation begins. It all starts with your beliefs.

Breast cancer survivors are among the smartest and savviest women I have ever met—not because they search the world over for the wisest doctors or uncover the most exotic treatment, but because they look within. And they start this inner journey with an unblinking examination of their beliefs about life.

The belief shift starts with the illness itself, challenging three widely held beliefs that work against overcoming breast cancer:

1. A diagnosis of breast cancer means my certain death.

2. The treatment of breast cancer is drastic, is of questionable effectiveness, and involves many side effects.

3. This diagnosis *just happened* to me, and therefore there is little I can do to influence it.

As you already know, all the above beliefs are untrue! But let's be certain we know the truth about these statements when they may appear. Here is the reality:

1. Breast cancer, no matter how advanced, may or may not mean death.

2. A wide range of breast cancer treatments do exist and have the potential to be effective. The benefits in recovery far outweigh the difficulties.

3. Most cases of breast cancer do not *just happen*. And your ability to influence your health is significant.

Knowing these truths will serve you well in your recovery. Your response to breast cancer is the central issue. Thankfully, there is much you can do.

The mind has a powerful impact on the body. Our beliefs affect the way we perceive illness and literally control our response to it. Beliefs determine emotions, which have a direct link to physical health. In short, our beliefs about ourselves, our disease, our treatment, and our role in healing are inextricably linked with outcomes.

> *Our beliefs about ourselves, our disease, our treatment, and our role in healing are inextricably linked with outcomes.*

Consciously and unconsciously, your beliefs are creating your reality. It's true, both positively and negatively. After interviewing more than sixteen thousand cancer survivors, I know of no survivors who believed that they could not get well. I also have observed that survivors come to understand that beliefs are just a thought. Thoughts can be changed. If we can bring ourselves to see the central role of beliefs, we can then create self-fulfilling prophecies based on nonlimiting beliefs.

Do beliefs affect recovery? Consider this. Beliefs and expectations constantly contribute to actual experience in all areas of life, including the experience of breast cancer. If we believe a rainy day means gloom, gloom is what we experience.

I fully realize it's a long way from rainy days to recovery from breast cancer. But this much is clear: Beliefs can be chosen. The sad fact is we seldom consciously choose them. Perhaps beliefs have simply been accepted by us for many years, like the conventional wisdom surrounding cancer. Perhaps we had beliefs imposed from parents, coworkers, or friends. We may have picked up other people's beliefs and made them our own. They may or may not be true or helpful. Yet these beliefs hold very significant power.

Awareness of our fundamental beliefs is often the first and certainly one of the most dramatic ways to improve our circumstances. If you are harboring the belief that breast cancer means death, I ask you to examine and challenge it. The fact is, there are long-term survivors of every type and stage of breast cancer, including many patients who have been told by doctors that there was no hope.

An Essential Thing You Can Do

Carefully analyze your beliefs. In your Wellness and Recovery Journal, complete the following sentences with the very first thoughts or feelings that come to mind:

1. I believe my breast cancer diagnosis means _____.
2. I believe my breast cancer treatment is _____.
3. I believe my role in survival is _____.

Now, please stop for a few moments and sit with these beliefs. Analyze how your beliefs align with truth. You may wish to talk to others who have successfully traveled the breast cancer journey. Understand what they believe. Vow to change any self-limiting beliefs today.

#31

Reframe Breast Cancer

If you're like many breast cancer patients, you look upon your illness as perhaps the most overwhelming threat to your life you've ever encountered. "My diagnosis was a force of evil," shared Carolyn. "I initially imagined breast cancer as my imminent demise, the certain end of my earthly existence."

Carolyn's words describe her mental outlook. Breast cancer . . . a force of evil . . . my imminent demise . . . the end of my earthly existence.

Beliefs like this call for a reframing. And one of the best ways to reframe is to come to view breast cancer not as a threat but as a challenge. In Carolyn's case, and after just a couple of counseling sessions, breast cancer became something that stimulated her toward introspection, to review her life. Carolyn ultimately made changes in her exercise routine, diet, vocation, and spiritual life. Breast cancer became her wake-up call.

Use the simple techniques of reframing throughout your life.

I am encouraging you to do the same. I ask you to move beyond the treatments for breast cancer and reframe this illness. In fact, I am asking you to use the simple techniques of reframing throughout your life. This means engaging in the process of finding alternative ways, more positive means, of viewing and responding to any circumstance.

Maria Walsh's diagnosis of breast cancer was the most frightening and unwelcome event in her fifty-eight years. Even though tests confirmed that the cancer had been discovered early and the prognosis was quite optimistic, Maria's chronic panic-driven thought process focused on her death. "I didn't just have cancer; I was cancer," she explained.

Jeannine Lobo also had breast cancer, but hers was significantly more advanced than Maria's. Jeannine had metastasis to the lymph nodes. Unlike Maria, Jeannine made the critical distinction that although she had cancer, the cancer did not have her. "I realized that my mind and spirit had cancer only if I allowed it." Jeannine's outlook reframed the cancer.

Jeannine's response demonstrates the significant power we possess. The point of control is not the circumstance of illness; it is our response to the illness. Our response can make all the difference. When we reframe breast cancer, we respond differently and more proactively. We acknowledge and nourish our inner strength, even in the face of doubt and fear. The threat subsides. We take on the challenge.

When we reframe breast cancer, we respond differently and more proactively.

Fortunately, both stories have happy endings. Maria was able to embrace many of Jeannine's more positive beliefs. Today both women are doing well.

An Essential Thing You Can Do

Examine your core beliefs. Then follow this reframing process, writing your answers in your Wellness and Recovery Journal:

1. What belief about breast cancer do I want to change?

2. What does holding this belief currently gain me?

3. How might I come to view breast cancer as an inspiring challenge rather than an overwhelming threat?

Reframe breast cancer. See it as a challenge that inspires you into action.

#32
Evaluate Your Self-Talk

Have you become mindful of the Voice, the presence in your head that carries on a constant conversation? From the moment we awaken in the morning until we drift off to sleep at night, we experience a continual stream of mental chatter. And when you are dealing with breast cancer, your self-talk can be nearly all negative and chock-full of fear. It makes for a terrifying life experience.

Marion Bricker called Cancer Recovery Foundation in a state of panic, her mind reeling out of control. After the first couple of minutes, I began to jot down the opening phrases of her sentences. They gave a clear picture of her state of mind:

"The cancer is spreading . . . I think my insurance is going to be canceled . . . How am I going to pay for this? It's all such a burden . . . I'm afraid of chemotherapy . . . My husband can't deal with this . . . I feel so frightened . . . Why did this happen to me? Where is God when you need him? There's nothing I can do."

Yes, there was something Marion could do! She could choose her thoughts. And you can, too. Believe it or not, we absolutely do choose our every thought. We may think the same fear-filled thought over and over, out of habit, but we are still responsible for that original choice. Analyze the thoughts you have been holding about breast cancer. That self-talk is the seed of your current experience of illness.

One of the most inspiring people whom I have encountered is Louise Lafferty. Lou is a woman who has every excuse needed to lead a life of despair. Childhood abuse, a turbulent early marriage, children in trouble, a toxic divorce, a child who ran away, a second husband who died in a work accident, a serious auto accident after which she was disabled for eight months, and then cancer. "My mind," explained Lou, "was always filled with thoughts of life being unfair and difficult, a battle."

Then Lou discovered this great truth: self-talk can change life.

Lou made massive changes. First, she came to the profound realization that her troubles were all in her past, over and done. What happened in the past did not automatically predict what would happen in the future. Of primary importance, Lou came to realize that the thoughts and words she chose right here and now were the ones creating her future. Her self-talk set in place her experience, either good or bad.

That was eleven years ago. I just heard from her over Christmas. Today Lou is cancer free, a happy, healthy, and whole person.

An Essential Thing You Can Do

Complete this awareness builder. In your Wellness and Recovery Journal, write down a positive, empowering message you can give yourself in the following circumstances.

Circumstance: You're frustrated at the doctor for his arrogance, impatience with your questions, and the limited amount of time he spends with you.

Positive self-talk:

Circumstance: It's three a.m. and you're wide awake, consumed with thoughts and fears of suffering and self-pity.

Positive self-talk:

Circumstance: Your energy level is at an all-time low. You are tired and discouraged, questioning if you can take any more.

Positive self-talk:

Now I ask you to take a moment to notice what you are thinking. Is your self-talk negative or positive? Do you wish for your future to be an extension of these thoughts? If not, change. Yes, you can. I believe in you.

#33

Choose a Daily Affirmation

Affirmations are positive statements of intent and belief. They take the place of the negative mental chatter, the self-talk that may be gripping you. Affirmations serve to *make firm* the positive things about you and your circumstances. They are consciously chosen self-talk.

Your words are constantly doing one of two things: building you up or tearing you down. So affirm positively. You are not so much changing the situation as you are changing your thinking about the situation. To be clear, affirmations will not cure your breast cancer. But affirmations will change your thinking about breast cancer and may be at the heart of experiencing wellness.

Affirmations will not cure your breast cancer. But affirmations will change your thinking about breast cancer and may be at the heart of experiencing wellness.

The constant conversation in our mind is processing everything; our internal dialogue is always interpreting events and creating meaning. Positive affirmations can guide and direct this inner conversation and, in the process, change our response. Affirmations are simply short statements that express the desired outcome. When combined with an acceptance that the old belief is changeable and the genuine desire to change, our affirmations begin to create a new reality.

Affirmations are most powerful when expressed in the present tense. The phrase *I am grateful for life today* is much preferred over a future-tense alternative *I will show gratitude for my life.*

Positive affirmations were first brought to notice in the Western medical world by Émile Coué, a 19th-century French pharmacist who noticed that several of his patients dramatically improved when they focused on positive health outcomes rather than on the negative fears and images of illness. Coué's famous affirmation, which he encouraged his patients to use, lives on today: *Every day, in every way, I am getting better and better.*

I realize affirmations can be difficult to believe. It's one of the central reasons that positive thinking is sometimes limited in its effect. An exclusive focus on the positive can result in a sense of unreality. As an example, if you have a strong inner belief that you are a bad person and disease is your rightful punishment, telling yourself that you are going to get well is probably not going to work. Predictably, it will be necessary to first recognize the underlying beliefs and challenge the negative ones before the positive ones can be effective.

Affirmation has been dismissed by many people in the medical community as brainwashing. In a way, it is. For years we may have been brainwashing ourselves with limiting beliefs such as "I am a bad person." When you substitute an opposite and nonlimiting belief such as "I am a child of God, worthy of all God's best," you are deliberately washing your brain with what may seem to be, at first, an artificial construct.

This artificiality is often a problem at first. For example, the affirmation "I am cancer free" sounds pretty ridiculous when you've just been given the negative results of a CT scan. But the key is to initially pretend, to play with the new belief as if it were true. Our minds cannot yet accept a belief that contradicts the old limits. But it can accept a kind of imaginary game in which we play with the new belief as if it were reality. And it is through this play and practice that the new belief gradually becomes believable.

In a spiritual sense, this is acting on faith. It's not that much different than the beliefs you act on when sitting down in a new chair. You seldom ask, "Will this chair hold me?" No, you assume it will hold you. In fact, you don't even question if it will hold you. You just sit down.

Likewise with a new belief. You begin to believe that your new belief can become reality, and so you act as if it is. At first you do this in very small ways, setting easily attainable goals. After time, the new belief becomes a way of life.

I changed my health with one very powerful affirmation. Right in the middle of the cancer battle, starting at the point where I was down to 112 pounds, confined to bed, and on morphine to control the pain, I began to affirm:

"I am cancer free, a picture of health."

I coupled this spoken affirmation with mental pictures of healthy pink cells, a smile on my face, and my body being vital and alive as I held my hands outstretched over my head. If you came to my home today, you would see a photo of me on my favorite beach, hands lifted overhead, greeting a new day, and affirming a new and healthy life.

This affirmation stirred a new belief. I would repeat it countless times—three hundred, four hundred, even five hundred times a day. I'd whisper it. I'd say it in a normal tone of voice. I'd shout it out loud—at least when no one was at home. I believed it. I acted on that belief. I credit this work of speaking health and healing into my life as the point of power that helped turn the tide in my cancer journey.

Change your mind, and you'll change your health. Affirmations can drive this process.

I am asking you to make affirmations work for you. Change your mind, and you'll change your health. Affirmations can drive this process. Whatever you affirm tends to become manifest in your life. Why not affirm the very best? Not out of a naïve blindness to illness, but out of the well-founded hope of creating your own positive self-fulfilling prophecies of health and healing.

Here's how I encourage you to challenge beliefs and make affirmations work for you:

1. Understand and accept that the old belief is not reality.

2. Nurture a genuine desire to change.

3. Substitute the old belief with the new affirmation.

4. Combine the positive affirmation with positive action.

An Essential Thing You Can Do

Study the following examples. Implement them in your own healing program.

Limiting Belief #1

Breast cancer means death. Similar beliefs: Cancer cells are powerful. I am always ill. My body is weak. My resistance is low. I might struggle, but the cancer will eventually get me.

Nonlimiting Affirmation

Breast cancer is a message to change. Similar affirmations: Cancer cells are weak and confused. I have a healthy body. I am building my immune function. My body has its own inner healing wisdom.

Limiting Belief #2

Cancer treatments are toxic and ineffective. Similar beliefs: I hate my treatments. I always get sick after treatment. I am always so tired after radiation.

Nonlimiting Affirmation

I have designed a treatment program that has my enthusiastic belief. Similar affirmations: I believe in my minimally invasive treatment choices. My treatment side effects are readily managed. I am filled with healing energy.

Limiting Belief #3

There is really nothing I can do. Similar beliefs: I am a victim of cancer. I have no control over what happens to me. I can't help what I think. I can't help what I feel. I have no choice.

Nonlimiting Affirmation

I control my response to breast cancer. Similar affirmations: There is a great deal that I can do. I am in charge of my own life. I have many choices. I have great creative resources.

Limiting Belief #4

I am afraid. Similar beliefs: I am helpless. I am trapped. I fear surgery . . . chemotherapy . . . radiation.

Nonlimiting Affirmation

I am filled with hope. Similar affirmations: I am confident. God's spirit of love is within me. I have positive choices.

Limiting Belief #5

I don't have energy. Similar beliefs: It's too hard for me. I am lazy.

Nonlimiting Affirmation

I am vital and alive. Similar affirmations: I have positive energy. Joy and pleasure help me heal.

Limiting Belief #6

This is going to turn out badly. Similar beliefs: I'm unhappy. There's no hope. I don't deserve healing.

Nonlimiting Affirmation

This experience is going to turn out perfect. Similar affirmations: I am happy. Life is good. I am worthy of healing. I accept myself as I am now.

Limiting Belief #7

I am a weak person. Similar beliefs: I am emotionally . . . intellectually . . . physically . . . spiritually weak. I am not capable of self-healing.

Nonlimiting Affirmation

I am a strong woman. Similar affirmations: I am filled with heart. I am filled with self-respect. I have a fighting spirit.

Limiting Belief #8

I'm not good enough in God's eyes. Similar beliefs: I'm not worthy. I'm not acceptable to God. I am always wrong . . . guilty . . . inferior . . . a failure. God is out to get me.

Nonlimiting Affirmation

God deeply loves me. Similar affirmations: I am a good person. God created me. I am a child of God. I accept myself as I am. I respect myself.

Limiting Belief #9

My doctors don't care about the real me. Similar beliefs: People don't really care. Healthcare professionals are only out for what they can get. My doctor rejects me. My doctor cares only about his fee.

Nonlimiting Affirmation

People like and care for the real me. Similar affirmations: My doctor did what he did with the best possible motives. He really does care for me. I care for myself.

Limiting Belief #10

Things will never get better. Similar beliefs: Things never change. Things are getting worse. I can never change. People in my life can never change. I'll never have the healing I want.

Nonlimiting Affirmation

Every day, in every way, I am getting better and better. Similar affirmations: Everything is changing for the better. My healing goes well. I feel good about myself. God is for me. Life is good. This day is good. I am worthy of all God's blessings.

#34

Manage Your Toxic Stress

Toxic stress is emotional overload, a sometimes-expressed but mostly suppressed negative overflow. Toxic stress is not the circumstances we are experiencing. It is the perception with which we are processing our experience. These perceptions are experienced in our mind independently of the circumstances. Importantly, these perceptions are under our complete control.

Toxic stress adds to the physical and mental anguish breast cancer brings. Stress works at cross-purposes to health, putting the mind in a state of confusion, blurring the focused peacefulness needed for healing.

There is something you can do about this perception. It's called the relaxation response. First named and described by Herbert Benson, MD, a cardiologist and associate professor of medicine at

Stress works at cross-purposes to health, putting the mind in a state of confusion, blurring the focused peacefulness needed for healing.

Harvard Medical School, the relaxation response is a simple, effective, self-healing meditation technique for reducing the detrimental effects of all kinds of stresses of everyday life, particularly stress associated with a life-threatening illness.

Benson found that the relaxation response is even more effective when one chooses a focus word or phrase that is closely tied to one's spiritual beliefs. The idea is to pick a word or short passage that has meaning for you: a Christian might use *The Lord is my Shepherd* from the twenty-third Psalm; a Jewish person might choose *shalom*; a non-religious phrase, such as the word *peace*, might be used.

Pick a phrase with significant personal meaning. Dr. Benson calls this the faith factor and explains that it can greatly contribute to helping our minds manage stress more effectively.

The quest for daily self-renewal starts with a decision to handle our problems with a sense of equanimity. Eliciting the relaxation response, especially when coupled with the faith factor, results in our minds working for, rather than against, our healing.

An Essential Thing You Can Do

Triggering the relaxation response is simple. Try these steps:

1. Find a quiet place, free from distractions, and sit in a comfortable position.

2. Pick a focus word or short phrase that is deeply rooted in your spiritual beliefs.

3. Close your eyes and relax your muscles, from toe to head, particularly relaxing the shoulder and neck area, where most tension is carried.

4. Breathe slowly and naturally. Repeat your focus word silently as you exhale.

5. Assume a passive attitude. When a distracting thought comes to mind, simply dismiss it and return to your focus word.

6. Practice this response for ten to twenty minutes twice a day.

7. In your Wellness and Recovery Journal, check your daily schedule. Do you have time blocked, twice a day, for stress management? Schedule it. Honor these appointments.

#35

Visualize Health and Healing

An extension of the relaxation process is visualization, also known as mental imagery. This is a valuable tool for helping you reinforce belief in a desired outcome. It is an extension of the relaxation exercises in that it is typically added at or near the end of the meditation period.

The essence of visualization is to first create mental pictures of your immune system and of your chosen treatment effectively fighting the breast cancer. You then visualize the breast cancer disappearing and your body returning to health.

Visualization is that simple; there's no need to make it any more complicated. I ask you to try it.

Consider some of these guidelines: Picture the cancer in symbolic images. For those who require a realistic image, you may want to consult an anatomy text to find pictures of actual cancer cells. Most patients, however, use symbols. I've had people describe their cancer as sand, a lump of clay, and even ice cubes. I saw mine as jelly. The most important criterion for picturing the disease is to think of the cancer as weak and confused. Don't give it power. Whether you visualize your cancer symbolically or realistically, what is important is the meaning you give it: visualize the cancer as weak.

Whatever the problem, give your body the command to heal itself, visualizing the process in a way that makes sense to you. End the imagery by seeing yourself well, free of disease, and filled with energy.

Imagine your treatment as strong and powerful, damaging only the weak breast cancer cells. Imagine your healthy cells remaining intact. Picture your immune system fighting the cancer. Imagine the weak and damaged breast cancer cells being naturally flushed out of your body. Picture the breast cancer shrinking until it is gone.

If you are experiencing pain, picture your white blood cells flowing to that area and soothing the pain. Whatever the problem, give your body the command to heal itself, visualizing the process in a way that makes sense to you. End the imagery by seeing yourself well, free of disease, and filled with energy.

How has this benefited you? Most people's fears tend to decrease as the imagery process gives them a greater sense of control. Ongoing research leads us to believe the imagery process has an influence on the body, actually triggering a hormonal and biochemical response to a renewed sense of hope. The resulting changes to the body's chemistry influence immune function, thus assisting the body in maximizing its opportunity to heal.

Visualization is controversial. More than a few healthcare professionals consider it to be a form of self-deception. "After all," they reason, "I can show you that the tumor has been growing."

I encourage you to consider this response. In your own mind, separate what is happening from what you wish to be the outcome. It is possible, and beneficial, to picture the breast cancer shrinking even though it may, at this moment, be growing. This is not self-deception. It is self-direction, and it's necessary to beginning the pursuit of any life goal. At first, reality will lag behind the vision you have of the desired outcome. But that vision will tend to pull us in the direction we need to go.

This is not self-deception. It is self-direction, and it's necessary to beginning the pursuit of any life goal.

How can you make this technique work for you? After evoking the relaxation response, try this:

1. Picture your cancer cells as weak and confused.

2. Create a mental image of your treatment and your immune system overcoming the cancer.

3. Imagine your body's natural processes eliminating the disease from your system.

4. Envision the cancer shrinking until it disappears.

5. Imagine yourself well, filled with vitality for living.

An Essential Thing You Can Do

Study the sample scripts in Appendix 5, "Meditation and Visualization." Choose one. Evoke the relaxation response. End it with a visualization exercise. Do so at least twice daily.

#36

Maximize Mind, Body,
and Treatment

Thankfully, conventional breast cancer treatments are becoming more targeted and affecting fewer healthy cells. But the fact remains, treatment side effects are the bane of the breast cancer journey.

Vitally important is the mind's role in combating side effects. In an experiment of a new chemotherapy, part of the group was given saline solution, sterile salt water, as a placebo. Fully 30 percent of this group lost their hair! It is common for patients to experience nausea, not during or after treatment, but on their way to treatment, known as anticipatory nausea. Add to this the legions of examples in which the same treatment results in radically different side effects for different patients, and what do you get? Even allowing for physiological differences, the mind is at work; our beliefs are turned into biological realities.

Two women may perceive their cancer treatments entirely differently. During one of our workshops, I asked Carol, a nursing home administrator, to draw a picture illustrating her body, her breast cancer, and her treatment. A few minutes later, she returned with a drawing of a huge devil injecting a charred and smoldering breast with a large syringe of poison.

At that same seminar, Rhoda told us that she initially refused chemotherapy because she saw it as poison, more deadly than cancer itself. When I asked Rhoda to draw a similar picture, she returned with drawings of chemotherapy as acid eating through a tabletop.

If you believe mind affects body, the implications of these images are significant. Negative perceptions of treatment stand in the way of the body's ability to respond favorably. Whenever a patient sees treatment as a friend, this positive perception starts to work beneficially with the treatment. The best way to make treatment a friend is to make certain you "own" the treatment program, knowing that this is what you consider to be the very best course of action at this time.

Your mind is the key. I want to help you program yourself for the most positive outcome possible by using a type of visualization that athletes have successfully employed in training. After evoking the relaxation response, picture yourself sitting in a chair or lying on a table having your treatment administered. In your mind's eye, see the cancer shrinking. Feel your strength returning. At the end of your imaginary treatment, envision yourself as vital and alive, ready to enjoy the gifts of renewed health and greater well-being.

If you do this frequently, especially during your course of treatment, evidence suggests your body will respond to the actual treatment with maximum capacity and minimal side effects. Like an Olympic athlete, you will be living the event in your mind first. Your mind helps the body get the message as to how it is expected to respond in the actual situation.

An Essential Thing You Can Do

View your treatment as a friend. Take time, make time, to imagine your treatment dramatically helping you. Envision yourself as well, free of any treatment side effects, and returning to radiant health.

....

Take a Break

The steps in this section are basic and fundamental mind-body principles. There's much more to healing with the mind. You may want to continue your training with more reading, seminars and workshops, and perhaps personalized instruction. But for the moment, I suggest you take a break from this work and do something that brings you joy.

The Sixth Step on the Incredible Journey:
Embrace Your New Life

Let breast cancer transform you. It is perhaps difficult to imagine any benefit coming from the experience of breast cancer. With the frightening diagnosis, the myriad of treatment decisions, and the need to manage all the potential side effects, how could breast cancer ever be a force for good?

Hundreds of thousands of survivors tell of the real and lasting changes that come directly from their breast cancer journey. A whole new and better chapter of life has opened before them. I wish this for you, too.

#37

Understand the Message of Illness

When you reframed breast cancer, you began to see illness as more of a challenge than a threat. Now I invite you to take this exercise one step further.

The challenge in illness can be found in its message to change. In a very real sense, the message of breast cancer is a call, an opportunity, for personal growth. In this reframing lies the seed of healing and well-being.

Could breast cancer be a message signaling you to make changes in your life? We've already suggested several on the physical level—diet, exercise, and lifestyle issues. Might there be more?

Many survivors come to the point where they view breast cancer as a call for personal transformation, to become a new person. The changes can go well beyond health habits and may lead to a profound personal awakening. The wise patient uses the experience of breast cancer as a turning point, a time to replace ineffective and limited ways of coping with healthier, more effective methods: nurturing relationships, developing vocational aspirations, and pursuing spiritual growth.

As soon as I suggest this position, people cry, "On some level, you're suggesting I gave myself breast cancer!" Not so! You clearly did not purposely set out to give yourself a serious illness. Don't read blame, self-sabotage, or guilt into the message of illness. Instead, realize the changes are potential points of power. If you and I may have participated in our illness, even subconsciously, then we can participate in our wellness.

Don't read blame, self-sabotage, or guilt into the message of illness.

I encourage you to explore the hidden messages of breast cancer. Many women discover a link between their physical, emotional, and even spiritual states of well-being and the onset of their illness. More important, many women trace the beginning of their healing to their decision to change these beliefs and behaviors. They were able to examine the deeper message in illness and choose a response that changed their lives.

If this analysis has interest for you at this time in your journey, start by asking yourself the following questions:

- What high-stress events or changes happened in the year or two prior to diagnosis?

  Become keenly aware of uncontrollable misfortunes. Death of a spouse or child, loss of a job, and financial setbacks are obvious candidates. Also include internal stresses, such as disappointments, major life adjustments, and ongoing conflict in important personal relationships. Many survivors can identify one or more major stress points in their lives prior to the onset of breast cancer.

- What was my emotional response to these circumstances?

  Did you process your grief over the loss, express your emotions, and finally adopt a hopeful stance? Or did you sink into a chronic depressed state? This is a measure of your participation. Don't read blame here. Participation simply refers to how you responded to the circumstances that may have triggered the stress. Might you have put others' needs before your own? Did you give yourself permission to mourn a significant loss, or did you determine you were going to be invincible and show no emotions? Did you permit yourself to seek the support of others during these stressful times? How effective was your emotional self-care? Many survivors gain significant insight from a close examination of these questions.

- How might my reactions to stress and loss be changed?

  Are there alternative ways of responding? Could these toxic circumstances and relationships be removed from your life? If not, how can you balance them, honoring your emotional needs first?

Give yourself permission to define your true needs. This is highly important work in health and healing. It is perfectly acceptable to find constructive and uplifting ways to meet these needs, regardless of what others may say or think. Give yourself that permission. Understand the message breast cancer has for you.

An *Essential Thing You Can Do*

Conduct a thorough and unflinching personal inventory. In your Wellness and Recovery Journal, complete this exercise:

1. High-stress events that occurred in the year or two prior to diagnosis or recurrence included _____.

2. My major emotional responses to these high-stress events were _____.

3. I could have changed these circumstances by _____.

4. I could have changed my emotional response by _____.

· · · · · · · · · · · · · · ·

Take a Break

Take another break. Complete the inventory and then stop your wellness work for today. Carefully contemplate the implications of the important issues raised in this exercise. You may wish to revise your responses after a time of reflection.

#38

Live Now

"Now" is such a wonderful gift. Many women with breast cancer needlessly miss it. "Now" is lost by living in the past or in the future. Instead, I suggest one of our shared goals should be to live well with the only time we do have—this very precious present moment.

How many times have you heard yourself say the following: "If only I hadn't done such and such. If only I hadn't smoked. If only I'd taken better care of myself. If only . . . If only . . . If only . . ." We mire ourselves in the regrets of the past and miss the moment we have been given.

At other times we get caught in the fear of the future. "What if the cancer spreads? What if the chemo fails? What if . . . What if . . . What if . . ." Here we miss the present moment because we are consumed with what may happen in the future.

Natasha Washington was diagnosed with breast cancer at the age of fifty. "I was consumed with worry," she said, "not just over my cancer, but about my elderly mother, who lives with me and my son. She is so frail. When I am at work, I feel as if I need to check on her several times a day. And what if she has to go into assisted living? How will I ever pay for that? Plus my alcoholic ex-husband keeps coming back into our lives. Why is he so weak? He was so mean to me. I feel like a complete failure. And now breast cancer."

Live now.
Live today.
Live this hour.

The answer: present-moment living. Live now. Live today. Live this hour. All our regrets about the past, no matter how sincere, won't change history. All our worries about the future won't add even another minute to our lives. On the contrary. Both fears and worries diminish our current moments.

In over a quarter century of this work, Bob Otis from Cincinnati, Ohio is the only male breast cancer patient I have personally met. He was diagnosed at the age of thirty-six. "[The cancer diagnosis] came just two years after buying a new home and the birth of our second child. But all I could think of in those two years was my failing sales career. Times are still tough. Our family's income is falling at the very time our expenses are rising. I just put the house on the market. There will be a loss. And now I'm looking for a new job. I feel so bad that the family has to suffer."

Natasha and Bob share a similar problem. Both are contaminating their present moments. Natasha's worries about the future ensure that she will enjoy little peace in this moment. Bob's life is consumed by regrets that imprison him in the past. Neither is living now.

Yet their only chance to capture health and healing is found here and now. What is required is a shift in thinking from what Bob might have done differently in the past or what may happen to Natasha in the future. Both will be better served when they focus on what each can do in this precious present moment.

Health, healing, and happiness are not completely dependent on our body's physical condition. High-level wellness is possible even with disability. I ask you to appreciate the fact that, even with breast cancer, you have life, here, now. Living each moment fully is the master secret to well-being.

Living well is a state of mind that has everything to do with the quality of our time. Living well is about this moment. Please, don't put off living a full life until you are physically "cured." Now is the time! This is your moment!

So with loving tenderness I ask, "What about you? Might similar shifts be required?"

Our potential for knowing well-being depends, in large part, on our ability to understand that the past does not equal the future. The past is over. Regrets, remorse, and recrimination cannot touch us unless we allow them to remain in our lives. The future cannot harm us unless we create a future based on perceptions of fear, anger, and guilt. The only time that contains the power to change our lives is this present moment. And just because you have breast cancer now does not predict with any degree of certainty that you will have it next year.

An Essential Thing You Can Do

Each day, I ask you to relinquish any thoughts or judgments that bind you to the past. Give up any fears that keep you from creating a healthy future. Choose one activity this day, this moment, that brings you pleasure, contentment, and happiness. Do it now! Know that the supply of these moments is limitless, there for the taking if you only choose to take them. Here, in the present moment, you will find your health and healing.

#39

Take Time to Play

My mentor was the late Dr. O. Carl Simonton, the father of modern psychosocial oncology. One of his landmark presentations was called "The Healing Power of Laughter & Play." Prior to one session at a natural-health conference, he had prepared three pieces of cheesecloth for each registrant. This light, airy fabric would readily float when tossed into the air.

Once distributed, Carl explained, "Now I am going to teach you to juggle." And in a matter of less than five minutes, he had twelve hundred people juggling cheesecloth. The sight was hilarious. People were overjoyed and laughing out loud. Even people who were struggling with illness were up on their feet, big smiles on their faces.

Finally, Carl asked everyone to stop juggling and then posed a fascinating question: "Will those of you experiencing pain at this moment please remain standing? Everyone else, please sit down." Three people remained standing. Three out of twelve hundred! Carl then explained the natural pain-reducing effects of our endorphins.

How much time have you allowed yourself for play in the last week? If you answered, "None," you are a member of a very large club. That's unfortunate. Living well requires play.

It's a common phenomenon. Most adults react negatively to the idea that we need to play. In fact, millions of people believe that grown-ups should not play. Somehow we think that playing is not the mature thing to do. If you are counted among this group, I ask you to challenge your thinking. From this moment forward, understand that play is an important part of your "work" of creating health and healing!

Understand that play is an important part of your "work" of creating health and healing!

The need to honor our playful nature is very strong. Most of us just repress it. Please don't. Give yourself permission to play, actually scheduling playtime in your daily calendar if you must. Treat that time carefully, assigning it the same importance and priority as other areas of life, such as work and family.

Analyze your own life. Have you noticed that you're never too tired to play? In fact, if you think you're tired, perhaps that is just the signal that you need more play. Play builds energy reserves; it is a major contributor to health and healing.

You and I were not put on the planet just to work, work, and work. We were created for joy. So create some joy in your life—play. Consider this list of ten noncompetitive activities:

1. Stroll on the beach.
2. Fly a kite.
3. Swim.
4. Ride a bike.
5. Draw a picture.
6. Write a poem.
7. Skip around the park.
8. Sing.
9. Listen to music.
10. Take the scenic route.

An Essential Thing You Can Do

Make your own play list by recording it in your Wellness and Recovery Journal.

....

Take a Break

Now, right now, I want you to stop reading, put aside this book, and go play for thirty minutes. Go! Have some fun. Do it! We'll continue creating health and healing a little later.

#40

Laugh to Foster Healing

Norman Cousins made many contributions to our understanding of the mind's role in mobilizing the body's healing processes. But none is so vividly remembered as his emphasis on laughter. In his 1979 book *Anatomy of an Illness*, Cousins called laughter "internal jogging." Since that time, science has confirmed that even something as simple as a laugh or a smile carries with it a positive biochemical response.

Since that time, science has confirmed that even something as simple as a laugh or a smile carries with it a positive biochemical response.

Lighten up! It will directly enhance your well-being. Just notice how relaxed you feel after laughing at a good story or watching a funny movie. It's wonderful!

In my home video collection, I have a surefire laughter generator. It's a series of DVDs called *The Best of Carson*. I realize that some of you are too young to remember that Johnny Carson was the king of late-night television. But he was host of *The Tonight Show* for thirty years. His ribald humor, unforgettable characters, and myriad of special guests put a smile on millions of faces at the end of every weekday. This DVD series has all the great moments. And no matter how many times I have seen it, I laugh until tears come to my eyes.

Please allow me my favorite Carson story:

An eighty-five-year-old man becomes engaged to marry a twenty-five-year-old girl. Thinking he may need a physical exam, the man makes an appointment with his doctor and shares the good news of his upcoming nuptials.

Surprised, his doctor says, "I want you to be very careful. Too much sex can kill a person."

The old boy pauses thoughtfully for a moment and finally replies, "Well, Doc, if she dies, she dies."

For most of us, seriousness is seen as an important virtue. Gravitas, we call it. We tend to think that laughing or giggling is childish behavior and certainly not appropriate for adults. I observe way too many cancer patients going through life with this fearful, beaten, and downtrodden seriousness surrounding them.

There is nothing inconsistent about being an adult and including laughter in your life. There is nothing wrong with being ill and pursuing a lighthearted approach to wellness. This is not some demented form of personal denial. Instead, it can be the opportunity to let the hidden child in you come out once in a while. Get in touch with that exuberant, vibrant part of yourself. Enjoy playing with your own children or grandchildren. And above all, please laugh at yourself and your seriousness.

An Essential Thing You Can Do

Go ahead. Rent that comedy DVD. Watch your favorite sitcom. Go to the local comedy club or a silly movie. Laugh! Let those positive biochemicals loose. It's healing.

#41

Evaluate Your Relationships

You and I constantly interact with other people—a husband or a wife, a friend or a lover, a child or a relative, a boss or a coworker; the list of our relationships is endless. At times, our lives seem to center entirely on relationships. How we get along with the significant people in our lives seems to determine, to a large extent, the quality of life we have. Furthermore, the absence of relationships can cause much disharmony and deep dissatisfaction. Like it or not, relationships are central to our experience of life and even our experience of healing.

Breast cancer survivors invest time and energy in relationships that nurture them. And survivors put relationships that are toxic on hold. Patricia shared in a support group meeting what this meant to her. "I had to move out. It was difficult, particularly leaving my two children. But I knew it was what I needed at that time. And I stayed away for nearly three months."

Patricia married while in college. She went to work to support her husband and his education. Patricia was expecting her first child before her husband graduated from dental school. She never earned her degree, something her husband seemed to hold over her.

"He was always criticizing me," Patricia said. "And I would yell back, trying to defend myself from attack. I'd bring up times when he disappointed me. And he would counter with a litany of my shortcomings. It became a vicious cycle. I had to leave."

Was a marriage gone askew partly responsible for Patricia's cancer? I believe so. Toxic stress lowers our resistance. Sadly, Patricia's search for love led to one affair and then another. Her guilt became overwhelming, leading to clinical depression. It wasn't long before Patricia was starting each day with a couple of vodkas in an attempt to numb the pain.

She came to believe the breach in her marriage was linked to her physical problems. After beginning her breast cancer treatments, Patricia finally began to look at the relationship with her husband.

I credit Patricia with wanting the relationship to work. With the help of a marriage counselor, she was able to better understand her part in the ongoing battles. She recognized her reactions and began to select different, more measured responses to her husband's remarks. Today, Patricia and her husband are working on improving their relationship. She is cancer free.

Our relationships with others reflect the relationship we have with ourselves.

I realize the sensitivity of this next statement, but please allow me to share a key insight you can use to your tremendous benefit: our relationships with others reflect the relationship we have with ourselves.

Do you experience conflict with a coworker? Look within to understand the inner conflict you may carry. Does a child seem self-willed and impossible? Look within: do you carry a belief that kids are willful and impossible?

Please don't interpret this as blame. I simply want you to know that your self-perceptions are exceedingly powerful and dramatically impact your relationships. When we evaluate relationships, the first task is to look at ourselves, discovering the truth: the only way to change another is to change ourselves first.

And the quickest, most certain way to change oneself is to switch from being a critic to becoming an encourager. This much is true: whatever you send out will always come back to you. If we criticize, note how we will be criticized. But when we encourage, note how encouragement is returned. Change and improve your relationships by sending out love, joy, and peace. Be an encourager.

Do healed relationships always equate with healed bodies? I know the two certainly correlate, but I can cite only anecdotal evidence. But when we heal our most important relationships, we are then free to move on to a healed life of our own. Simultaneously, we create a relationship environment that often corresponds to vast and rapid physical improvement.

An Essential Thing You Can Do

Conduct an inventory of the ten most important relationships in your life. Number a page in your Wellness and Recovery Journal from 1 through 10 and record the people's names. Did you even realize these were the ten most important people in your life?

> *The quickest, most certain way to change oneself is to switch from being a critic to becoming an encourager.*

Highlight any relationships that need to be put on hold. Are there any that need improvement? Indicate those. What is one thing you could change that would improve each relationship?

Come back to this list often. Keep it current. Declare any relationship war to be over! Affirm that you now live in joy and peace. Appreciate how important this work is to your health and healing.

#42

Get Beyond "Why?"

It's the inevitable question breast cancer patients ask: "Why did this happen to me?"

The trouble with the "why?" question is that we seldom like the answers we are given. In fact, we fight the answers, not wanting to accept. Some think breast cancer is entirely a lifestyle issue: "She ate terribly and was way overweight." Lifestyle may be the cause for some, but the reason does not stand up to scrutiny for all breast cancer patients. Others say the "why?" is environmental: "We've polluted the planet. We're all getting sick." That may explain some cases, but why is it that other people exposed to the same carcinogens remain perfectly healthy?

Religion tries to answer the "why me?" question. I've been told by well-meaning clergy that God was using cancer to punish my sins, to correct me for my eternal profit, to draw me closer to God, and to help me learn submission. Incredible!

When we ask "why," we are often looking for someone or something to blame. "Why?" is another way of saying we are helpless and the situation is beyond our control. Some cancer patients blame others, some blame circumstances, some blame parents, some blame doctors, some blame the environment, and some blame God. Affixing blame does not help. It only creates helpless victims, something I trust by now you believe you are not.

Here's my personal insight on this question. The road to personal wellness starts when we stop asking "Why?" and begin to consider the question, "Toward what end?" or "For

The road to personal wellness starts when we stop asking "Why?" and begin to consider the question, "Toward what end?" or "For what purpose?" Put another way, "How can I make this experience benefit myself, others, and the world?"

what purpose?" Put another way, "How can I make this experience benefit myself, others, and the world?"

Thousands of the cancer survivors I have interviewed speak of "God not being done with me yet." Could that be the case with you? Instead of asking, "Why me?" let's ask, "What can I be doing to be part of the solutions to the many problems in this world?" That single query is central to transcending the "why" of breast cancer.

An Essential Thing You Can Do

In your Wellness and Recovery Journal, start a new page with the heading "How can I make my experience of breast cancer beneficial?" Journal how you believe cancer can help you grow and be of service to the world. Refine this list as your insights deepen.

#43

Practice Gentle Self-Discipline

Living a life based on maximizing your well-being requires living with values and behaviors that may be radically different from the ones you had before your illness. Some days, the work of creating health and healing may not be easy or convenient. On a cold and rainy morning, it might be tempting to stay in bed and forget our morning exercise. And instead of preparing a high-nutrition lunch, it might seem simpler to use the drive-through window of the nearest fast-food restaurant. Our intention to move toward wellness may seem strong, but too often our practices may not reflect that intent.

I know. And I am a student of self-discipline, not a master. Just today I bought a chocolate bar. Now in my defense, it was dark chocolate, 70 percent cacao, the healthier choice. But I realize I cannot do that often and write about self-discipline with any degree of integrity.

See yourself as self-disciplined. Wellness self-discipline includes thought and deed, intent and practice. This principle is equally valid whether you are facing a just-baked batch of chocolate-chip cookies or a dark cold morning of exercise. There's no need to deprive yourself, just discipline yourself. That means one cookie, not the whole plate. That means at least a short walk rather than no walk. Gentle, wholesome self-discipline is at the core of making health and healing real in your life.

The issue is not whether we can choose health. It's whether we can envision ourselves choosing wellness. Remember: "The me I see is the me I'll be."

The issue is not whether we can choose health. It's whether we can envision ourselves choosing wellness. Remember: "The me I see is the me I'll be."

The practice of seeing yourself as self-disciplined leads to two very powerful life qualities: self-respect and freedom. When your walk matches your talk, when intent and action are one, you have a consistency in your life that is unshakable. You are grounded in a principle-oriented life experience, firm in the knowledge that all you are doing physically, emotionally, and spiritually is in your best interest.

Envision yourself as happily self-disciplined. Inner strength and self-respect flow from this position. The discipline to actually act on what is important to you leads to personal freedom; you are no longer bound by the traps of obsession, compulsion, and self-pity. This is a personal power at the highest level, a strong and quiet inner assurance that is one of the rewards of successfully traveling the breast cancer journey.

"But I am just not a naturally disciplined person," protested a young woman during a question-and-answer session we held in London. Of course she is right. None of us are naturally self-disciplined. It's all about choice.

The issue becomes which habits we will choose in our lives. I am asking you to choose positive addictions like healthy diet, daily exercise, and more. The result is self-respect and freedom.

An Essential Thing You Can Do

Match your walk with your talk, your actions with your best intentions. Choose one area—perhaps diet or exercise—and make that your focus today. For example, for one day excel at maximizing your nutrition. Then choose another area for the focus of the next day. And another the next. Feel your self-respect skyrocket. Congratulate yourself. Bask in the personal power and freedom this discipline brings to you.

44

Choose Your Emotional Style

What is your dominant style of expressing emotion? Is it suppression, in which you constantly restrain yourself from venting real feelings? Or overreaction, in which you are too exuberant or you fly into inappropriate rage? Or denial, in which you tend to push feelings out of your consciousness? Or have you found the balance, in which your emotional expression contributes to your health and healing?

Two raw emotions concern me most: fear that is denied and hostility that is either suppressed or overexpressed. Our goal here is to become a skilled observer of our emotions and to learn the ability to choose the best and most appropriate responses.

You have the right to feel any emotion. Any and every emotion you feel is perfectly acceptable. We're human; we feel. In a real sense, we are emotionally driven creatures. One moment we're angry; the next moment we're sad. We're happy and we laugh. The next moment we're fearful of some loss.

I've observed that people tend to repeatedly experience four basic emotions: mad, sad, glad, and egad—anger, depression, happiness, and fear. All of them are acceptable.

Health-enhancing emotional processing can be easily summarized by the phrase review, release, and renew.

To experience an emotion, and recognize that any emotion is perfectly normal, is one level of understanding. But the healthful processing of those emotions is quite another. It's here we typically find our challenges.

Health-enhancing emotional processing can be easily summarized by the phrase *Review, release, and renew*.

Review the emotion. The most damaging mistake we make in emotional expression is to attach too high a priority on either burying or venting the feeling. Instead, start by observing the emotion. Review it. Understand it. That's half the challenge.

Then release the emotion. Get rid of the anger, the sadness, the fear. It's perfectly acceptable to feel the way you feel. It's your emotion, and you own it. But then release it in a nonhostile way, without being coy, subtle, or vague. Think or say, "I'm upset, but it's only my emotions. It's over and done. Life goes on." Release.

Then renew. Think and say, "I can choose my emotions. My emotions do not choose me." You then replace the emotion. Consciously choose a more loving, more spiritual response.

This process is exceedingly powerful. For example, my personal emotional challenge is effectively processing anger, one of the most highly charged emotions. My anger is generally short-lived, a negative emotion over a single event. When I'm functioning at my best, I'll review it: "There's my anger. I recognize it. It's starting to boil my water." Then I'll release it: "Anger, go away. I become upset when you're around." I express it, without malice. I release it.

The trouble comes when I don't renew, when I fail to consciously replace that anger with love, or at least compassion. When I fail to replace anger with love, I find myself walking through a field that is filled with land mines. The slightest nudge, and an explosion erupts. Not until I review, release, and honestly renew can I master my emotions.

You possess this same ability. Renewal is actually very simple. For me it comes when I focus my attention on what actually provoked me. If I will just reflect on the event, I will often discover that I perceived the provoker—be it a person, event, or condition—with fear. I was the one who was fearful that my person, property, or pride was under attack.

This is a profound discovery of the highest importance in our healing, one that affects us on every level of our lives. It's fear we are dealing with, actually our perception of fear. That perception is under our control. Once we understand and observe our fear, we can review, release, and verbalize that fear. "This diagnosis scares me." Or "Doctor, I reject that prognosis." Thereafter, we can renew by substituting a more hopeful emotional stance.

One of our workshop participants wrote in her evaluation, "You helped me become keenly aware of my emotional style. Simply observing the situations that trigger my emotions allows me to rethink my perception that I am always under siege. Instead of perceiving fear, I can now understand the situation in the light of compassion. This is a new and miraculous emotional insight, one that immediately begins to dissolve my resentments and helps me immensely in my healing."

Make it your priority to become a keen observer of your own emotions. Review, release, and renew. It is the secret to emotional well-being.

An Essential Thing You Can Do

Become an objective observer over the next week. When an upsetting event occurs, record the event in your Wellness and Recovery Journal. Then record your emotional response based on one of three categories: denial ("I denied that there was any problem"), suppression ("I suppressed my emotions when I really wanted to tell that person off"), or overreaction ("I went crazy and overreacted, way out of proportion to the whole event").

Learn the new three Rs: review, release, and renew. You'll become a skilled observer of your own emotional stance toward life. Reactions and emotions that were once automatic will now come under your control. Through it all, you will achieve new levels of well-being.

> *Learn the new three Rs: review, release, and renew.*

The Seventh Step on the Incredible Journey: Nurture Your Spirit

I trust you have been following and implementing the steps in this book. If so, you are well on your way to triumph over breast cancer. Once again, you can do this. I believe in you.

Many cancer survivors go even further, reaching for higher levels of well-being in all areas of their lives.

"I see [cancer] as a gift," says singer Olivia Newton-John about her journey through breast cancer. "I know it sounds strange. But I don't think I would have grown in the areas I did without this experience."

This is the promise of transformation in the breast cancer journey. It's there. Join me now in continuing our quest.

#45

See Life through Spiritual Eyes

What do you see when you look at your life? Do you see a body riddled with disease, dreams hopelessly derailed, a family frightened, and a life lived in despair?

Or can you see a precious moment, a special instant in space and time when mind and spirit are ill only if you allow it? Are you able to grasp the beauty and grace, even the perfection, in your life without coloring those qualities with the pain of breast cancer or the hurts of life?

One of the most courageous and gracious women I had the privilege of meeting was Elizabeth Edwards. She was an activist, author, breast cancer spokesperson, political wife, and, most important, mother. Elizabeth saw life through spiritual eyes. Her example is an inspiration for all who are on the incredible journey.

Like you, Elizabeth's life was filled with both joy and pain. Hers was often magnified because she and her family were frequently in the news. Elizabeth's joy centered on her family—four children, one of whom, her son Wade, died in an automobile accident.

For thirty years, she was married to John Edwards, a successful attorney-turned-politician and one-time presidential hopeful. But after her breast cancer relapsed, it was learned that her husband had a sexual relationship with a videographer. He later admitted to fathering a child with the woman.

Elizabeth's pain ran deep. Even though they separated, she refused to diminish her husband in the eyes of her children. She wrote them a letter as only a mother could do. Elizabeth guided and encouraged them with messages like "You don't know when your time is up. Do today what you want to accomplish. And strive to end each day by being able to say, 'This day was well spent.'"

Just one day before losing her battle to breast cancer, Elizabeth wrote a message on her Facebook page. "You all know that I have been sustained throughout my life by three saving graces—my family, my friends, and a faith in the power of resilience and hope," she wrote. "These graces have carried me through difficult times, and they have brought more joy to the good times than I ever could have imagined."

Elizabeth's memorial service was held in the same church as her son Wade's. The nation mourned her passing. But to this moment, we are blessed by her life.

Elizabeth Edwards lived life from both the head and the heart. For her, life was ultimately a spiritual journey. She saw the larger picture, and it made her life a living legacy from which we all can learn.

I am encouraging you to also see life through spiritual eyes. Spiritual eyes allow us to see the value of what is simple and readily available in spite of the circumstances in which we may find ourselves.

"I awoke from my surgery," wrote Pontea Kamal, "and there in my room was my husband. He was holding our little daughter, propping her up on the hospital bed. And she was squeezing my finger. Her big dark eyes looked at me, and she smiled as she said, 'I love you, Mommy.' It was such a precious moment. Now, since my breast cancer, I see life much more clearly."

Join me in a commitment to no longer dwell on what is wrong or to take inventory of what is missing. Let's put our focus on all that is right, all that we have.

Join me in a commitment to no longer dwell on what is wrong or to take inventory of what is missing. Let's put our focus on all that is right, all that we have.

This level of awareness brings a vastly different experience of breast cancer. Embrace this consciousness. There are miraculous moments in your life right now—each and every day. Appreciate them.

An Essential Thing You Can Do

I ask you to pause and spend a few moments to see life in a more spiritual light. Ask yourself, "What do my countless blessings really mean to me?" This new awareness may contribute more toward your well-being than the most potent medicine.

#46
Value Personal Spiritual Growth

Too many people equate victory over cancer with a doctor's report that says, "This patient is clinically free of any sign of cancer." I understand that desire, I share that desire, and in fact, my records state exactly that. I wish you the same. But that is not the most important part of the journey. For the person who opens his or her mind and spirit, the cancer experience evolves into a transcendent spiritual journey.

You may say, "Greg, I'll settle for a cure. Just get my life back to normal." Don't settle for that! Remember, you don't want things to get back to normal. In fact, after your experience with breast cancer, things will never be the same again. You want a new and better life. It comes in the form of a new spiritual walk.

Breast cancer has pounded you with a million hammer blows. But you have the last word as to how those blows will shape you. William James, the distinguished psychologist and philosopher, declared that his generation's most important discovery was that human beings, by changing their inner attitudes of mind, could change the outer aspects of their lives.

By making personal spiritual growth our aim, the most important outcome will be to use the experience of cancer to shape us into wonderfully different creatures.

I see you changing in that way, using the hammer blows of breast cancer to change your inner state of spirit. By making personal spiritual growth our aim, the most important outcome will be to use the experience of cancer to shape us into wonderfully different creatures. Indeed, cancer can reshape our attitudes, soften our spirits, and transform our lives.

It's personal spiritual growth we seek. Think of spiritual growth as the natural and logical extension of your healing journey.

First, you made the decision to do everything possible to get well again. Next, you devoted time and energy to understanding your treatment options, to improving your diet, to daily exercise, to making positive beliefs and attitudes real in your life, and to nurturing your most important relationships.

Now, in a seamless progression, I am inviting you to explore and develop your own practices of gratitude, forgiveness, unconditional love, and more. It's the spiritual part of the healing journey—the most important part.

Cynicism has no place here. You cannot climb up the spiritual mountain by thinking downhill thoughts. If you feel that life is filled with despair, that it is now gloomy and hopeless, and that spiritual growth is impossible for you, I ask you to challenge those thoughts. We must change our inner world before we can change our outer world. When you do, I can attest that healing awaits you.

Associate with people who are walking the spiritual path. This may mean some of your relationships change. But know that your spiritual journey can be advanced by cultivating relationships with those who have a spiritual vision.

In your own way, pray. Be still. Listen to the still, small voice within. It's the quiet, positive, and hopeful voice telling you what to do and what to be. Don't beg or plead. Just listen.

An Essential Thing You Can Do

In your Wellness and Recovery Journal, record one spiritual quality that you would like to make vivid and real in your life. I began mine with forgiveness. Practice that quality for just one hour. Then extend the time. Keep this as your central goal. Quiet your mind and spirit. Listen. Act.

#47

Make Forgiveness a Way of Life

Forgiveness saved my life.

After I was told by my surgeon that he thought I had about thirty days to live, I was put in touch with an exceptional breast cancer survivor who kept prodding me to examine the issue of forgiveness. Her name was Colleen, and she was convinced that healing and forgiveness are inextricably linked. After weeks of resistance, I took her counsel to heart.

It didn't take me long to recognize what was at the core of my unforgiveness. My father and I had a toxic and tumultuous relationship. The only communication we had when I was a youngster was his profanity-laced epithets criticizing literally everything I did or did not do. During one frightful incident, I was convinced he was only seconds away from murdering me. The memory still puts fear into my heart.

Colleen's repeated warnings about unforgiveness led me face-to-face with my deeply buried anger toward my father. After some extended reflection, I came to see him as a product of his own abusive alcoholic father. And my father was plagued with his own demons, spending time in a mental hospital.

In a way, he didn't have a chance; he simply didn't know any better. And once I comprehended that fact, I was finally able to release, let go, and forgive.

Forgiveness is essential to getting well and staying well. Unless there is a healing of our mind and our spirit, any healing of the body is incomplete, and we are likely doomed.

Today I share Colleen's belief that forgiveness is essential to getting well and staying well. Unless there is a healing of our mind and our spirit, any healing of the body is incomplete, and we are likely doomed.

You may say, "Greg, you don't understand. Forgiveness in my case is just too difficult. The past is simply too horrific. People hurt me beyond forgiveness. My hostility is justified. I will not let it go."

When we embrace that attitude, the only person we are hurting is ourselves. Unforgiveness is like a red-hot coal we hold in the palm of our hand. We are the only person it is burning. Let's be clear: We're not forgiving for the other person's benefit. We're forgiving for our own benefit, releasing the toxic poison that contaminates our life.

In as gentle and sensitive a spirit as I can communicate, I am asking you to search your heart for any sign of unforgiveness. You'll very likely find somebody, or a whole list of people, who has done you wrong. If so, you will help in your healing by releasing thoughts of resentment, recrimination, or remorse.

Forgiveness is work that brings with it huge rewards. Forgiveness links our newfound awareness of the sources of health and healing with our awakened understanding of our emotional style. The promised benefit is the emotional and spiritual peace we need for healing.

This is a big promise. Forgiveness keeps the promise.

I believe forgiveness, when it actually becomes a way of thinking and living, is the single most powerful key to a healed life. Forgiveness is a trusted technique by which our thoughts and perceptions are changed, transforming the harmful effects of toxic emotions into the healing reality of compassion, even love. Forgiveness allows us to switch our focus from fear to love; it helps us change what can be changed and allows us to make peace with the rest—a profound dimension of healing.

Forgiveness allows us to switch our focus from fear to love; it helps us change what can be changed and allows us to make peace with the rest—a profound dimension of healing.

Opportunities to learn and practice forgiveness are everywhere. The obvious teachers of forgiveness come in the form of people, most often individuals who antagonize us, the ones whom we can't stand to be around.

Just as important as forgiving others is being self-forgiving. Let's be honest, we often hold much resentment and shame against ourselves. We don't let go easily. In the quiet moments, we judge ourselves harshly, "I'm so stupid. I'm fat. I'm ugly. I'm not worthy. I probably deserve this illness." The list is without end.

Like never before, this is the moment to release that self-condemnation. The only way is through forgiving yourself.

Let go. I observe so many cancer patients carrying self-concepts of unworthiness. These are false and deadly beliefs. Yes, we may have done something undesirable, but that is our behavior and does not equate with being an unworthy person. Release those feelings of shame.

A young single mother shared, "I was a drug addict and a prostitute. Now cancer. But I think I deserve it. God is punishing me."

"No," I responded. "Absolutely not! Release those beliefs. They are serving only to condemn you to a life of dis-ease. Forgive yourself. Forgive others. Ask God to forgive you. Release it all."

There's also judgment. Our critical perceptions of others create a battleground of emotional turmoil. It is so easy to judge others. Judgmental behavior tears at the fabric of relationships and kindles the fires of resentment. Breast cancer is, among other things, an opportunity to learn and practice the difference between acceptance and approval and thus to transcend judgment.

Like never before, this is the moment to release that self-condemnation. The only way is through forgiving yourself.

I urge you to practice acceptance. A couple came to our offices. She had breast cancer, and her husband had prostate cancer. They soon began to tell the tale of their son who was gay. While the woman was accepting; the man was not. There was so much strife between the father and son—fights, accusations, condemnation. The son left for college and never returned home. For more than six years, the two hardly spoke. It weighed so heavily on the father. Then his cancer diagnosis.

"I knew that forgiveness and reconciliation were central to my getting well again," said the man. "I finally reached my son on the phone and said I would like to see him. When we met, the first thing I promised was to never again mention his lifestyle."

Forgive. Let go. Release. Yes, forgiveness is the answer. All of us have imperfect natures. All of us exhibit behaviors that don't match our potential. We all miss the mark. Forgiveness allows us to accept imperfection without having to approve of it.

Forgive. Let go. Release. Yes, forgiveness is the answer.

I have noticed that not everything in life meets my expectations. You may have the same experience. But we can find peace through acceptance. Only forgiveness brings personal peace that is the rich soil where health and healing take root.

Forgiveness is experienced on two levels. The first is the most obvious. There is an event: We are wronged or we perceive an attack. That behavior needs to be forgiven. When we can say, "I forgive myself for _____," or "I forgive _____ (another) for _____," then we have embarked upon the forgiveness journey.

The second level of forgiveness changes our perception of what happened. Yes, an event occurred. But the real problem starts when we begin to judge what happened, when we label ourselves or the other person as bad, hurtful, mean, stupid, or another unkind attribute. We perceived the event as unfavorable; the event didn't meet our approval. We judge, even condemn.

The alternative? Acceptance. Accept ourselves. Accept others. Accept that life happens. It's part of being human. Forgive and accept. It is a far better way to live.

People who are, or believe themselves to be, near death often come to the realization that forgiveness heals. Feuds, differences, and deep hurts suddenly seem less important at this time.

Marilyn Ellis, in the middle of a battle with cancer, felt terribly ill at ease when her mother and father visited. Marilyn and her mother would make noble efforts to get along with each other, but they seldom fully succeeded. Old patterns of attack and defense were constantly cropping up between them. Childcare, cooking, homemaking, religion—the particulars didn't seem to matter. Her mother wanted a more conservative daughter. Marilyn wanted a more enlightened mother.

"It was driving me crazy," said Marilyn. "During her last visit, I was ready to throw her out. But then it occurred to me, God isn't looking at my mother and thinking, 'Mildred is such a bitch.' How could I pretend to want to get along with my mother if I was so consumed by my judgment of her?

"So I said to myself, 'I'll try this for an afternoon. I'll focus on acceptance and give up approval.' From that moment, the situation and the relationship started to shift. As I was more accepting of her, she became more accepting of me. We're a long way from spiritual soul mates," conceded Marilyn, "but there is a stronger growing bond between us."

Perhaps you struggle with hidden hostility and resentment. The amazing payoff of forgiveness is that so many people do get well after letting go. Lives are certainly made better; many are made longer. But it strikes me that if one is willing to forgive during the last moments of life, why not do it earlier? Like right now?

How often do we need to forgive? Always. Don't drag the memories of past hurts and mistakes into your present moments. Nothing from the past is important enough to allow it to pollute our present. Let go of judgment. Nurture compassion. You deserve it. You'll change your life—forever!

How often do we need to forgive? Always. Don't drag the memories of past hurts and mistakes into your present moments.

Forgiveness was the absolute turning point in my own cancer recovery journey. I can trace the exact time of regaining my physical strength and emotional well-being to an intense week of sincerely forgiving others and myself. And from that point forward, I have attempted to make forgiveness a way of life.

How about you? Might forgiveness have a place in your journey?

An Essential Thing You Can Do

Choose just one hurt and forgive everyone concerned with it. Say out loud, with complete sincerity, "(Name), I totally and completely forgive you. I release you to the care of God. I affirm your highest good." And in the same way, forgive yourself.

Feel the warmth of forgiveness. This next week, choose one person to forgive each day.

#48

Exude Gratitude

What is the least healthy habit, the one that causes dis-ease of every kind? It's ingratitude—the lack of thankfulness, our inadequate appreciation for the great life we enjoy. The practice of gratitude is central to the healing process.

Even with breast cancer, even in the middle of a difficult treatment cycle, even in your darkest and most fearful hours, I am encouraging you to be thankful for all you do have. For life, for love, for family, for friends, for the awesome beauty of nature, for all these things and more, be thankful.

Why do I feel so strongly about gratitude's healing power? It's because I have seen gratitude bring more significant and rapid improvements in the lives of cancer patients than any other single action. Yes, I do mean that literally—more significant than surgery, more than radiation, more than chemotherapy. Gratitude is the physiological spark that sets the healing process in motion. I am urging you to be grateful.

> *I have seen gratitude bring more significant and rapid improvements in the lives of cancer patients than any other single action.*

If you wish to cultivate a deeper attitude of gratitude, I suggest you begin to see yourself as a guest who is only visiting here on earth. All that you have is not really yours; it is a gracious gift from your host. During your stay, you are privileged to enjoy the gifts of friends and family, home and transportation, food and recreation, vocation and service. Even your health, no matter what the state, is another of those gifts.

Jill Phillips lay near death in a small rural Nebraska hospital after being told she was "filled" with cancer and that it was inoperable. Mired in despair and self-pity, she could see nothing for which she could be thankful. "I was divorced, my two children were grown and lived in different parts of the country. I hated my dead-end job. My life seemed miserable.

"But one night I looked out of my hospital window to see a deep, dark sky that was filled with stars. I shut off all the lights in my room and just gazed at the sky for what must have been hours. I started to ask a lot of questions: 'What is this huge universe all about? What is my place in it? Why am I sick?' I can't say I received a lot of answers. But I did discover a new perspective.

"I became thankful," continued Jill, "grateful just for being a part of this huge and wonderful world. I realized that in my fifty-plus years, I had been able to experience so much. The marvel of giving birth to two other lives—what a miracle! The beauty of the country, where I feel such strong roots; I was so grateful to live here rather than in a city. The deep friendship I had with my sister—I was so thankful for her love. That night at the window changed my whole perspective on my problems. Yes, I have cancer. But even more, I am grateful."

Like Jill, we too can capture true well-being when we choose gratitude. But so many roadblocks on the cancer journey seem to detour us, to mire us in ruts of ingratitude and self-pity. We're so busy with appointments and treatments, discomfort and despair, fear and pain, that we lose our perspective. We tend to look at the cancer journey as a long and twisted path, filled with deep potholes. There seems to be nothing for which we can be thankful. I suggest we see this outlook as faulty and self-destructive thinking.

I also suggest that each and every day you join me in declaring your gratitude. My daily affirmation is "I am so happy and grateful now that I am healthy, blessed in every way."

Yes, I really do speak that declaration every day. And I believe it sets a tone that helps create my reality.

Exude gratitude. It transforms the very experience of illness and of life. See beyond the daily challenges of breast cancer, the worries that seem so all-consuming. Treasure the wonder of life. Become aware of your guest status in this brief moment in time and space. Be thankful. It heals.

An Essential Thing You Can Do

It's time for another page in your Wellness and Recovery Journal. Complete the following sentence:

"I am so happy and grateful now that _____ _____."

Express your gratitude—every hour of every day.

#49

Practice Unconditional Loving

Loving heals. Even though there may be times when we are lost in the abyss of our physical maladies or buried in the agony of our emotional awfulizing, with each moment comes a new opportunity to choose loving. This is a decision that truly heals.

As I previously shared, I prefer the word *loving* over *love*. It denotes the action necessary to bring the idea of love to life. Love is not loving until it is released, until it is intentionally given.

Loving without condition is an intentional choice we make about what thoughts, words, and deeds are coming from us rather than coming to us. The choice to love means we don't have to wait for the medical test results, the doctor's assurances, the elusive remission, or the hoped-for cure. We can choose to love now, this moment—regardless of the circumstances. This choice heals.

I ask you to consider this perspective. The crippling fears surrounding breast cancer are actually the absence of love. This absence of love is like darkness that is merely the absence of light. You don't solve a problem of darkness by yelling at it or fighting it. If you want to get rid of darkness, you turn on a light. So it is with fear. Don't yell. Don't fight. Instead, turn on your love light.

I realize I am asking a lot. I understand this is a profound and radical call. Loving is more than a thin veneer. It is an act of heroism and courage of the highest order.

You should not seek or even expect accolades. Unconditional loving is not a decision surrounded by pomp and circumstance. Most often it has to do with small choices. "How do I choose to respond to this person? How can I best help another? How can I best nurture myself?"

On the surface, the conditions and circumstances of breast cancer do not easily inspire loving. Taken by themselves, these conditions and experiences often elicit fear, helplessness, and even despair. Face it, this incredible journey has many such moments.

But we can choose the loving response anyway! When we do, invariably the result is a renewed sense of hope that results in a strong biochemical "live" signal to body, mind, and spirit.

Loving starts with self-loving. Here's a hard-won insight that has taken me more than twenty-five years to fully grasp: We can know true healing only from a position of personal spiritual strength. And it is self-loving that is the wellspring of this vital force.

Do you love yourself? Do you believe in your self-worth? I hope you do. And I want to help you affirm your great value. In fact, right here, right now:

I declare that you are healthy and whole.

I declare that you are vital and alive.

I declare that you are strong and courageous.

I declare that you are discerning and wise.

And I declare you have all you need to survive and even thrive after breast cancer.

You are a great person. There is simply no way you cannot love the wonderful person you are. And know that breast cancer does not detract one iota from your self-worth. So please, love yourself. Look in the mirror, peer into the eyes of your soul, and say, "I love you." Self-loving. It's the root of recovery for thousands of patients.

Loving is the first and last word in healing, the great balm that quiets distress, the only real magic bullet against breast cancer, and the strongest vaccine to combat malignancy.

Our greatest enemy is not disease but despair. Unconditional loving is the healer.

An Essential Thing You Can Do

It is decision time once again. Decide to practice unconditional loving for the next hour. And the next hour, and the next. You will know healing—something far greater than a cure.

#50

Share This Hope

Now that you've invested time reading this book and following at least some of the steps, you're aware that there is much you can do to improve your well-being. Your choices and actions really do make an enormous difference in the journey through breast cancer. In partnership with your medical team, you are now on the pathway to creating health and healing.

But many people don't know these powerful truths. Or if they do, they have only a vague acquaintance, not a working knowledge. They deserve more.

Share this hope with others who have been diagnosed with breast cancer. Share it with those who wish to prevent breast cancer. Discuss these ideas. Encourage one another. Make it your new priority to walk the path toward healing with someone else. This has the cumulative effect of helping yourself while helping another.

I invite you to contact us. You may even decide to be one of our 1,000 Voices who are spreading the word of the Vitamin D Promise in communities nationwide. 1,000 Voices is a new program of Breast Cancer charities.

We also have a free e-newsletter for you, plus a variety of helpful wellness resources. Believe it: you have a caring partner in your journey.

An Essential Thing You Can Do
Contact Breast Cancer Charities of America at *www.thebreast cancercharities.org*.

⌐ Epilogue ⌐
You Have a Future

THIS IS NOT THE END OF A BOOK. It is the beginning of a lifetime journey.

While breast cancer is certainly a serious illness, anyone who has traveled this incredible journey knows that it is as much an emotional, psychological, and spiritual walk as a physical one. They also know what a meaningful contribution the mind and spirit can make.

Tap deeply into the mental and spiritual assets with which you have been endowed. Use illness as an opportunity for personal growth. At times, that may seem beyond the scope of your thinking. I believe that it can be accomplished. Illness has been the pathway for millions of people to discover an even better life than they ever dreamed possible. Illness can be your wake-up call, a chance to experience the life you may have been forced to put on hold.

No matter how much time you think you may have to live, make the decision to live today—fully! Make the profound choices to forgive and to love. This leads to a better life and, as thousands of us believe, a longer life as well.

Let this illness be your new beginning. Choose to be well this moment. A hopeful, happy future can be yours. Choose it now. It's truly the essential thing you can do when the doctor says, "It's breast cancer."

Appendixes

Food as Medicine

HIPPOCRATES, THE FATHER OF MODERN MEDICINE, said, "Let food be thy medicine and thy medicine thy food."

Following medical care, dietary changes are the most common—and effective—strategies adopted by cancer survivors. The increasing importance of nutrition to optimize recovery has been one of the most significant discoveries in the last decade of cancer research, and the fact that cancer remains much less prevalent in cultures that continue to eat the unrefined foods of our ancestors is significant.

In short, there has never been a more important time in your life to eat well. This series of appendixes contains sample menus; a guide to making over your kitchen pantry, refrigerator, and cooking style; and a sample shopping list of green-lighted foods. This is the information you need to help begin a nutritious lifestyle, thereby promoting healing and recovery.

Appendix 1
Sample Menus

COUNTLESS TIMES I HAVE BEEN ASKED for sample meal plans. I am pleased to offer here two variations with two options for each meal. With simple substitutions, you can create a joyful variety of delicious meals that maximize nutrition.

Breast Cancer Charities Sample Meal Plan:
Three Squares a Day
Meal #1

Option A:	Option B:
scrambled egg whites with red bell peppers and onions	oatmeal
tomato slices	soy milk
orange	blueberries
herbal tea	ginger tea

Meal #2

Option A:	Option B:
chicken caesar salad with whole-grain croutons	veggie burger
carrot sticks with hummus	whole-grain bread
iced green tea	mixed green salad
	fresh tomato juice

Meal #3

Option A:	Option B:
baked eggplant	wild salmon
whole-grain dinner roll	brown rice
steamed broccoli	cauliflower
mixed green salad	Greek salad
apple slices	fresh plum

Breast Cancer Charities Sample Meal Plan: Four to Six Mini-Meals a Day

Meal #1

Option A:	Option B:
fresh tomato juice	grapefruit
whole-wheat bagel with peanut butter	hard-boiled egg

Meal #2

Option A:	Option B:
mixed green salad	nonfat yogurt

Meal #3

Option A:	Option B:
vegetable soup	mixed green salad
cheese	almonds

Meal #4

Option A:	Option B:
protein bar (low-sugar)	apple

Meal #5

Option A:	Option B:
herb-encrusted fish	roast turkey breast
mixed green salad	cauliflower

Meal #6

Option A:	Option B:
nonfat yogurt	celery sticks with hummus

Appendix 2
Clean Out Your Pantry
and Refrigerator

L ET'S GET SERIOUS. Your refrigerator and pantry are likely to contain lots of processed foods. If ever there was a time to eat real food, breast cancer is it. Now I ask you to take a bold step toward making thoughtful choices about nutrition. Once you clean out the shelves, you're on your way to bringing health to your dinner plate.

Throw out the following oils:

- margarine
- solid shortening
- partially hydrogenated oil
- all products made with any of the above

Buy the following oils:

- extra-virgin olive oil
- nonfat vegetable oil spray
- sesame oil

Throw out the following sweeteners:

- sugar
- aspartame

- saccharin
- all products made with any of the above

Buy the following sweetener:

- stevia

Throw out the following meats:

- salami
- bologna
- sausage
- bacon
- hot dogs
- smoked ham
- smoked turkey
- all products made with any of the above

Appendix 3
Cook and Shop Healthfully

Healthful Cooking Methods:

- coat the pan with nonfat vegetable oil spray
- stir-fry
- oven-fry
- bake in parchment or foil
- poach
- steam
- stew

Season Healthfully Using Herbs and Spices

To flavor:	Use:
vegetables	basil, caraway, chives, dill, ginger, oregano, rosemary, tarragon
fruits	cinnamon, cloves, mint, nutmeg
meats	curry, dill, fennel, garlic, oregano, parsley, rosemary, sage, tarragon, thyme
salads	basil, chives, dill, marjoram, mint, parsley

When you shop:

1. Read labels.
2. Buy choices low in fat, salt, and sugar.
3. Eat before you shop.

Appendix 4
The Real Food Shopping List

The Breast Cancer Charities Shopping List
Feel free to copy this list and bring it with you to the market.

Vegetables	Fruit
___ broccoli	___ berries
___ cabbage	___ oranges
___ peppers	___ grapefruit
___ tomatoes	___ mangoes
___ carrots	___ apples
___ leaf lettuce	___ cherries
___ cauliflower	___ apricots
___ onions	___ cantaloupe
___ beets	___ kiwi
___ asparagus	___ pears
___ squash	___ red grapes
___ pumpkin	___ watermelon

Fish and Meat

___ cod

___ flounder

___ tilapia

___ salmon (wild)

___ tuna

___ trout

___ mahimahi

___ sardines

___ haddock

___ skinless chicken breast

___ skinless turkey breast

Legumes

___ black beans

___ garbanzo beans

___ kidney beans

___ navy beans

___ pinto beans

___ lentils

___ split peas

Whole Grains and Breads

___ oats

___ oatmeal

___ barley

___ brown rice

___ flaxseed

___ buckwheat

___ spelt wheat

___ millet

___ amaranth

___ pita bread

___ wheat germ

Other

___ garlic

___ ginger

___ cinnamon

___ cayenne

___ stevia

___ green tea

___ curry

Nonfat dairy

___ yogurt

___ cottage cheese

___ almond milk

Oils

___ extra-virgin olive oil

___ sesame oil

___ nonfat vegetable spray

Complementary Treatment Modalities
Appendixes

YOU MAY DECIDE TO CHOOSE a complementary therapy to integrate into your healing program. There is excellent evidence that many mind/body/spirit approaches can play an important role in the healing process.

Meditation, for example, produces demonstrable effects on brain and immune function. Some of the side effects of conventional cancer treatments may be lessened with the integration of a complementary modality like acupuncture. Complementary modalities can also support healing by supporting your immune system and reducing pain.

Complementary modalities include a wide range of approaches. There are many opportunities to pursue these activities with a practitioner or by attending a class in your community. The approaches described in these appendixes are those that have been helpful to thousands of cancer patients around the world.

Appendix 5
Meditation and Visualization

FOR MANY OF US, OUR MINDS ARE SO BUSY with thoughts that we rarely create the opportunity to simply be at peace, relaxing into the present moment, quieting our minds, and being more aware of the sensations in our body.

By practicing meditation, which is simply learning to relax and be at peace, we can become more open and attentive to our deeper, intuitive wisdom and the healing potential that lies within us. By invoking this relaxation response, our body moves into the parasympathetic mode in which physical healing is optimal.

Meditation is a way of cultivating moment-to-moment awareness, and it supports becoming more present to our own experience. To do this requires that we become aware of the constant stream of thoughts and reactions to our inner and outer experiences in which we are all normally caught up. During meditation or contemplation, we discover that we are constantly generating thoughts and reactions. By simply becoming aware of our breath instead of the stream of thoughts, we become more aware of our body experience, allowing us to release pent-up anxieties and emotions. With practice, we can move toward acceptance and the release of stress and even limiting beliefs.

Meditation is a valuable way of reestablishing inner calmness and balance in the face of emotional upset or when you have a lot on your mind. We have all experienced how relaxing it can be to sit alone for a few minutes and just breathe, in and out, deeply and quietly, especially when life around us becomes stressful and out of balance. Research has shown that meditation can alleviate psychological and physical suffering of persons living with cancer.

Guided imagery is an extension of meditation. A leader or a recorded script is often employed to assist the participant in visualizing health and healing. Guided imagery has been credited with reducing side effects, pain, and stress. It can also aid in emotional coping with cancer and assist in preparing the patient for anticipated situations, such as surgery or chemotherapy. The imagery process can also be helpful in decision making and can be employed to improve mental health and control. Finally, guided imagery can reduce the need for pain medication. Research shows an increase in natural killer cell activity as a result.

Both meditation and guided imagery are less about method and more about calming your body and living in the present moment. By cultivating clarity and peace in meditation, by imaging health and healing, we become more accepting, less judgmental, and happier. What follows are some suggested scripts for your consideration.

Meditation and Visualization: Sample Scripts

Relaxation Exercise

Here is a simple exercise to help you to fully relax your body.

1. Close your eyes, remove your glasses if you wear them, loosen tight clothing, and take your shoes off.

2. Sit in a chair. Start by adjusting your position so that you are sitting comfortably. Don't cross your legs, ankles or feet, or hands. Sit with your back supported. If your legs are too short to reach the floor comfortably, then put a book or bag on the floor on which to rest your feet. Or lie on the floor if you wish.

3. There may be sounds in the room or outside. Try to ignore them. Remember that life goes on and that we can become relaxed despite the noises around us.

4. Raise your shoulders up to your ears and let them fall down gently.

5. Open your mouth as if yawning, close it a little, and rock your lower jaw left and right.

6. Close your mouth and push your tongue hard up to the roof of your mouth. Let the tongue spring back. Loosen your jaw more.

7. Once again, raise your shoulders to your ears, then release them gently.

8. Breathe normally and softly.

9. Allow your inhalations to become a little deeper.

10. As you breathe, just notice the breath and bring your attention to the sensation of the breath flowing at the tip of your nostrils.

11. Now notice the natural, gentle movement of your chest as you breathe in and out.

12. Take a deep breath without straining. Allow the breath to come and go effortlessly. Continue for a moment or two longer. Allow the natural rise and fall of your breath to help you to soften, relax, and remove any tiredness or tension.

13. As you breathe in, bring in softness and relaxation. As you exhale, take away any tiredness or tension. Inward breath brings softness and relaxation. Outward breath takes away tension.

14. Continue to breathe slowly and peacefully.

15. Check around your body. Is there any remaining tension or tiredness? If so, take your breath there to soften and renew.

Healing Meditation Exercise

1. Find a comfortable place to sit with your back straight and your feet firmly on the ground. Try to ensure that you will not be disturbed during your meditation—take the phone off the hook or turn the answering machine on.

2. Take about five minutes to relax your body completely, working from the feet up to the head. Imagine that you can just let

go of all the muscles; feel them soften and release, allowing the tension to flow out of your whole being. Focus particularly on the shoulders, neck, and jaw, as these are areas where we often, without realizing it, hold a great deal of tension.

3. When your body feels totally relaxed, bring your attention to your breathing. Don't change it. Just be aware of the breath moving in and out of your body.

4. Notice as much as you can about your breathing. How does it feel as the breath moves in and out of the nostrils? Where do you focus on leading your breath in your body? Stay with this for another five minutes or so.

5. Now imagine that you are outside in the sunshine. Get a sense of the light of the sun, warm but not too hot and shining down on you. You might like to imagine that you are lying on a quiet beach soaking up the sunlight.

6. Imagine that you can breathe in the light of the sun, taking it into your body. Let the light fill up every cell of your body. When you feel glowing and full of light, let that light move anywhere in your body where you feel you are in need of healing. Feel your cells transforming, becoming energized as the radiance heals and restores you.

7. Now let the light expand out of you. Radiate the light around your body so you are imagining yourself glowing with light and health. Stay with this part of the meditation for about ten minutes.

8. Now bring your attention back to the breath. Every time you breathe in, silently say, "I am breathing in health." And on each exhalation, say to yourself, "I am happy and whole." As you do this, feel the truth of what you are saying. Believe it so that it becomes a reality for you.

9. Now let it all go and bring yourself back to the room, slowly and gently. Feel the ground beneath your feet, and become aware once more of your surroundings.

You may wish to expand your meditation and visualization experiences. Many communities offer classes that can assist you in perfecting these skills. There are also many recorded meditation scripts that can be helpful in assisting your efforts.

Appendix 6
Yoga

GENTLE YOGA IS HELPFUL FOR PEOPLE dealing with illness, inviting them to listen and reconnect with their body. Through yoga, you will gain a greater understanding of how you can support your body in healing. Start with hatha yoga, which focuses on simple and achievable movements, focused breathing exercises, and relaxation techniques. I personally like the DVD series *Yoga for Beginners*, which is widely available where books are sold.

Appendix 7
Bodywork

THE TERM *BODYWORK* REFERS TO THE ARRAY of touch therapies that support balance and well-being. These techniques work because they deepen our mind-body awareness, which in turn allows us to let go of tension, release emotions, and support healing.

If you choose to explore one of these techniques, you may wish to first speak to a practitioner and discuss how they may be able to specifically support your needs. Ask questions such as "What happens during a session?" and "What benefits can I expect?"

Here are some of the most popular bodywork therapies:

Alexander Technique

Decreases muscle strain, nerve pain, chronic pain, fatigue, and post-surgical weakness.

Craniosacral

Treats muscle tension, injury, structural misalignment, and nerve dysfunction. Decreases stress.

Massage

Massage is the systematic manipulation of soft tissues of the body to enhance health and healing and can be used to achieve an improved level of well-being. From a medical or therapeutic perspective, massage can help a person living with breast cancer by reducing pain, anxiety, and stress and providing a caring touch.

Massaging the tumor itself is not recommended. However, people with breast cancer should not fear that massage is dangerous. In fact, massage can be a very important part of a complementary cancer care program.

There is no evidence to suggest that touch or gentle massage causes metastasis. But there is ample evidence that it greatly benefits many cancer patients, both physically and emotionally. In fact, touch addresses not only physical needs but also emotional, social, and spiritual needs as well.

Skilled touch can be beneficial at every stage of breast cancer treatment and recovery. Receiving comforting, attentive massage reminds us that the body can be a source of pleasure. It also can influence our ability to enjoy the present moment and feel our aliveness. A massage helps in reuniting body with heart, mind, and soul.

Excellent research has shown that massage can positively affect many cancer symptoms or side effects from conventional treatment regimens. These include nausea, fatigue, insomnia, and pain. Massage supports relaxation, which in turn supports immune function. Thousands of breast cancer patients report an increased sense of well-being and a reduction in anxiety and muscle tension.

Manual lymph drainage (MLD) is a safe, gentle massage technique that is used to treat many health conditions. It does not treat breast cancer itself but helps to improve symptoms of cancer treatments such as pain, neuropathy, lymphedema, scars, and postsurgical swelling.

Lymphedema is a condition that occurs in 30 percent of patients who have had breast cancer treatment. It is a swelling that occurs most often in the arms or legs. Lymphedema is a result of an impaired lymphatic system due to chemotherapy, radiation, surgery, or removal of lymph nodes. It can be managed or prevented with the timely application of combined decongestive therapy (CDT). This involves skin care, exercise, compression, and manual lymph drainage.

Polarity Therapy

Emotional and physical energy balancing. Improves circulation. Relieves pain and stiffness. Increases energy, flexibility, and clarity.

Rolfing

Deep-muscle bodywork. Decreases stress, chronic pain, and stiffness. Improves breathing, mobility, energy, and posture.

Shiatsu

Reduces stiffness, pain, fatigue, and stress. Improves energy and sleep.

Appendix 8
Energy Work

THE ENERGY IN OUR BODY IS SO NATURAL and spontaneous, we almost never stop to think about it. Thousands upon thousands of chemical reactions are taking place in the body at any one moment. Plus countless electrical impulses are passing through every part of our body. As well as having our own physical levels of energy, we are also part of the entire flow of energy around us.

The intricate network of energy in our body forms part of the energy of the natural world. We are each a miniature field, interconnecting with the electromagnetic energy of the world around us. By keeping our own mind-body-spirit in balance, we support our own well-being and contribute positively to the greater whole.

Therapeutic Touch

Therapeutic touch is often referred to as a form of energy healing or a subtle energy technique. It is directed to the energy field around the body, rather than with the muscle and connective tissue or with the physiological processes of the body. When practicing this modality, the therapist often does not touch the physical body but directs energy with hands positioned a few inches above the body. Therapeutic touch has been found to reduce stress, support relaxation, and promote healing.

Healing Touch

Healing touch is another method of energy healing that incorporates techniques that work directly on the body as well as on the energy around the body. The goal of this treatment is to align the body's energy and bring it into balance. Healing touch can create a deep relaxation, which supports the body's ability to heal.

Reiki

Reiki is a Japanese word referring to universal life energy. During a Reiki session, the practitioner's hands most often are in direct contact with the recipient's body rather than being held above, as in therapeutic touch.

Appendix 9
Naturopathic Medicine

NATUROPATHIC MEDICINE IS A SYSTEM of healthcare emphasizing illness prevention, treatment, and the promotion of optimal health through the use of therapeutic methods and modalities that encourage the self-healing process. Naturopathic practice blends centuries-old knowledge of natural, nontoxic therapies with current advances in the understanding of health and human systems.

Naturopathic diagnosis and therapy incorporates both traditional approaches and, increasingly, therapies supported by scientific research drawn from peer-reviewed journals from many disciplines, including naturopathic medicine, conventional medicine, European complementary medicine, clinical nutrition, phytotherapy, pharmacognosy, homeopathy, psychology, and spirituality. Clinical research into natural therapies has become an increasingly important focus for naturopathic physicians.

Naturopathic medicine:

- Acknowledges the healing power of nature
- Emphasizes disease prevention and encourages building health by assessing health risk factors and hereditary susceptibility to disease and making appropriate interventions to prevent illness
- Identifies, treats, and removes the underlying causes of illness, rather than suppressing symptoms
- Adheres to the dictum "First do no harm"; utilizes methods and substances that minimize the risk of harmful side effects;

avoids, when possible, the harmful suppression of symptoms; employs the least force necessary to diagnose and treat illness

- Acknowledges the role of doctor as teacher to educate patients and to encourage self-responsibility for health; honors the therapeutic value inherent in the doctor/patient relationship

- Treats the whole person

Naturopathic medical care can be utilized to help maintain the physical well-being of patients going through the various stages of a breast cancer treatment program. This includes both before and after chemotherapy, radiation, and surgery. Naturopathic medicine has been shown to alleviate the symptoms or negative side effects that often follow cancer treatment.

For patients who choose to explore targeted naturopathic cancer treatments, individualized programs are available. People who are in remission or cancer free and would like to improve their overall health and well-being can also benefit from naturopathic medical approaches. Pursuing detoxification while supporting health and immune function is an important cornerstone in naturopathic cancer care.

A naturopath may also employ the therapeutic application of air, water, heat, cold, sound, light, and the physical modalities of electrotherapy, diathermy, ultrasound, hydrotherapy, therapeutic exercise, and naturopathic manipulative therapy.

This may be accomplished by therapies including the following:

- Intravenous vitamin C
- Intravenous glutathione
- Intravenous hydrogen peroxide
- Chelation therapy
- Neural therapy
- Ozone therapy
- Colonics

- Constitutional hydrotherapy
- Hyperbaric oxygen therapy

In order to practice these specialized procedures, a naturopathic physician must undergo advanced training. Look especially for a naturopathic doctor (ND) with a degree from Bastyr University, the most esteemed naturopathic medical school in North America.

Appendix 10
Traditional Chinese Medicine

TRADITIONAL CHINESE MEDICINE (TCM) practitioners use methods such as acupuncture, herbal formulas, diet and lifestyle counseling, massage, and exercises such as Tai Chi and Qigong to restore the flow of Qi, vital energy, and the balance of yin and yang to the body.

TCM diagnosis is based on examination of the pulse and tongue as well as observation and extensive questions. TCM views health as a state of harmony and balance between mind, body, and spirit.

Chinese medicine developed from tribal roots. By 200 BC, traditional Chinese medicine was firmly established. Even though they did not understand the body in the way that modern medicine does, ancient Chinese physicians recognized that the body provides sensitive signals about health and the nature of illness. These signals are perceived as symptoms such as abnormal temperature sensations, altered thirst, increase or decrease in appetite, and changes in emotional states.

A TCM examination is thorough and noninvasive. The practitioner will take a careful family and personal medical history, noting your body's reaction to stress and stimuli such as heat and cold. She will observe the color and form of your face and body, note the condition of your skin and nails, look at your posture, and even listen to the sound of your voice. The condition of your tongue, including its shape, color, and coating, also provides important data on the way your circulation and metabolism is affecting your internal organs. Your pulse will be felt at three different points on each wrist, each location corresponding, in TCM theory, to a different part of the body. Considered together, this information gives the practitioner a sense of your body's current functioning.

Acupuncture is a branch of traditional Chinese medicine that involves inserting needles through the skin at specific points to treat various health problems. The classical Eastern explanation for how acupuncture works is that channels of energy, or Qi, (pronounced "chee") run in regular patterns through the body and over its surface. These channels, or meridians, are like rivers flowing through the body to nourish the tissues.

There are fourteen major acupuncture meridians, and each of these is believed to be associated with a particular part of the body. An obstruction or blockage in the movement of Qi creates imbalance and pain in the body and can lead to disease.

By manipulating the needles in a certain way, the practitioner attempts to bring energy to areas that are lacking or to create flow in areas that are blocked, bringing a sense of balance back to the body. Most people feel very relaxed during and after the treatment.

The National Institutes of Health Consensus Statement on Acupuncture concluded that acupuncture has been found to be a promising treatment to help ease the side effects of conventional cancer therapies such as chemotherapy and radiation. It can also be effectively used to control pain, improve quality of life, and strengthen the immune system.

TCM practitioners believe that in order for cancer to exist in the body, there must be certain factors and imbalances present to a greater or lesser degree. These factors include blood stagnation, energy weakness, phlegm, and other environmental toxins.

Acupuncture is also used by TCM practitioners in an effort to counterbalance the damaging effects of chemotherapy and radiation, thus helping the body to heal itself. TCM treatment may also help to support the immune system and digestive functioning.

In addition to acupuncture, a TCM practitioner may make recommendations on diet, exercise, herbs, and lifestyle modifications based on your current state of health and alter as needed.

Resources

YOU'LL WANT TO BECOME IMMERSED in mobilizing all your health and healing assets.

I ask you to study these resources, which are readily available where books are sold:

Anderson, Greg. *The Cancer Conqueror: An Incredible Journey to Wellness* (Andrews McMeel, 1990) and *Cancer and the Lord's Prayer: Hope and Healing through History's Greatest Prayer* (Jordan House, 2006). Two of my messages of hope and encouragement found through the body-mind-spirit connection.

Benson, Herbert, and Miriam Klipper. *The Relaxation Response* (William Morrow and Company, 1975). The definitive source for relaxation and meditation concepts and techniques.

Borysenko, Joan. *Minding the Body, Mending the Mind* (Bantam, 1988). How to manage stressful thoughts and uncertainty.

Lerner, Michael. *Choices in Healing: Integrating the Best of Conventional and Complementary Approaches to Cancer* (MIT Press, 1996). The intellectual's guide to alternative treatments.

LeShan, Lawrence. *Cancer as a Turning Point: A Handbook for People with Cancer, Their Families, and Health Professionals* (Plume, 1994). The emotional aspects of cancer. Helpful exercises involving reflection, discussion, and writing to help come to terms with fears.

Servan-Schreiber, David. *Anticancer: A New Way of Life* (Viking, 2008). Insights into healing by a professor of psychiatry and doctor who was diagnosed with a brain tumor.

Siegel, Bernie. *Love, Medicine and Miracles: Lessons Learned about Self-Healing from a Surgeon's Experience with Exceptional Patients* (1986, HarperCollins). Stories about self-healing from a former surgeon's observations of cancer patients.

Simonton, O. Carl, Stephanie Matthews Simonton, and James Creighton. *Getting Well Again: The Bestselling Classic about the Simontons' Revolutionary Livesaving Self-Awareness Techniques* (Bantam, 1992). Guides cancer patients to participate in recovery through imagery and therapy.

About the Author

"**A** MAN ON A MISSION . . . "
Greg Anderson is widely recognized as one of the world's leading wellness authorities. He is the founder of the Cancer Recovery Foundation International, a global group of affiliated charities and organizations whose mission is to help all people prevent and survive cancer.

Cancer Recovery Group focuses on integrated cancer care programs, improving the lives of all people touched by cancer. The affiliates also sponsor research into less toxic and minimally invasive cancer treatment.

Breast Cancer Charities of America (*www.thebreastcancer charities.org*) is the Foundation's newest and fastest-growing affiliate. It is the nation's first cancer organization whose programs are devoted exclusively to researching, educating, and delivering integrated breast cancer prevention and treatment protocols.

Greg Anderson was diagnosed with Stage IV lung cancer in 1984. His surgeon gave him just thirty days to live. Refusing to accept the hopelessness of this prognosis, he went searching for people who had lived even though their doctors had told them they were terminal. His findings from interviews with more than 16,000 cancer survivors form the strategies and action points for what has become an international cancer recovery movement. Anderson is widely recognized as one of the world's leading wellness authorities. He is the author of thirteen books, including *The 22 Non-Negotiable Laws of Wellness* and the inspirational classic *The Cancer Conqueror*.

To Our Readers

Handwritten note in top margin: "Red Mt Resort Utah St George"

CONARI PRESS, AN IMPRINT OF Red Wheel/Weiser, publishes books on topics ranging from spirituality, personal growth, and relationships to women's issues, parenting, and social issues. Our mission is to publish quality books that will make a difference in people's lives—how we feel about ourselves and how we relate to one another. We value integrity, compassion, and receptivity, both in the books we publish and in the way we do business.

Our readers are our most important resource, and we appreciate your input, suggestions, and ideas about what you would like to see published.

Visit our website, *www.redwheelweiser.com*, where you can subscribe to our newsletters and learn about our upcoming books, exclusive offers, and free downloads.

You can also contact us at info@redwheelweiser.com.

Conari Press
an imprint of Red Wheel/Weiser, LLC
665 Third Street, Suite 400
San Francisco, CA 94107